INTRODUCTION

Frankly with you, I ached to be an outgoing person for a long time. As a youth, I wished I could go to parties and have huge loads of energy to talk, associate, and appreciate meeting new individuals. On occasion, I even wished I could be the bubbling energy source everyone crowds around. I envisioned the number of more companions I would have and the amount more well known I would've been if by some stroke of good luck I might have been more outgoing. For sure, I begrudged outgoing individuals, and partially, may in any case begrudge them today.

There were on many occasions where I put forth a valiant effort to be pretty much as intriguing as conceivable just to be disregarded inside five minutes since I didn't have the energy to keep up with casual discussion. I would then become undetectable to the degree that it appeared to be trivial to have opened my mouth in any case. Have you at any point experienced anything like that?

I've ended up in discussions where I don't have anything to say more regularly than I'd prefer to concede. It happens most when I'm conversing with individuals from the other gender. It's somewhat weird. I read a ton and have a very capable of humor, however I can transform into a truly exhausting individual at parties.

Often, I would get back from parties feeling discouraged. I continued to think I should have been more intelligent, more appealing, seriously intriguing, and more alluring. It felt like I was never great enough.

At one point, I even Googled "how to turn out to be more interesting!"

Maybe you can relate child that? I used to rebuke myself for being to timid to mingle, and frequently pinned it on weakness. I developed to despise social butterflies for their capacity to keep up with discussions in noisy and occupied conditions. In spite of the fact that I knew attempting to turn into the energy everyone needs was close to incomprehensible, I was unable to let it be known to myself. This self-protection instrument might have been a way for me to abstain from resolving my concerns and accepting my actual personality.

Right away, I thought my issue was absence of certainty, emphaticness, or authority abilities. Albeit this was consistent with a specific degree, it wasn't the entire story. At that point, I didn't completely get what it intended to be a loner. In reality as we know it where extroversion appeared to be the standard, I was making a decent attempt to stop my self preoccupation. It ended up being an unthinkable assignment, yet it took me a surprisingly long time to understand that fact.

Action step

On a size of 1 to 10, how evident are the accompanying assertions? Rate yourself utilizing the workbook.

1. I disdain casual chitchat, however I appreciate profound conversations.
2. I get drained in case I stay at a party for too long.
3. I feel like all that I say ought to be significant and frequently avoid talking for this reason.
4. I favor one-on-one, or little gathering discussions over talking in huge groups.
5. I want to invest energy alone to re-energize my battery.
6. I think before I speak.
7. I experience issues thinking when in a gathering. I think best when I'm on my own.
8. I normally listen more than I talk.
9. I detest interruptions.
10. I disdain conflict.

Click on the link below to download your FREE action guide:

http://whatispersonaldevelopment.org/the-flourishing introvert

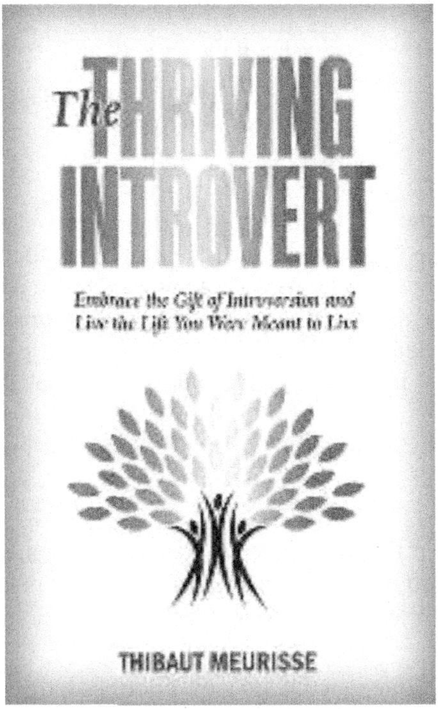

1

UNDERSTANDING INTROVERSION

> *What constitutes an introvert is quite simple. We are a vastly diverse group of people who prefer to look at life from the inside out. We gain energy and power through inner reflection, and get more excited by ideas than by external activities. When we converse, we listen well and expect others to do the same. We think first and talk*

later. Writing appeals to us because we can express ourselves without intrusion, and we often prefer communicating this way. Even our brains look different than those of extroverts.

— LAURIE HELGOE, AUTHOR OF INTROVERT POWER.

Many outgoing people fail to see being a contemplative person. It's difficult for thoughtful people to get outgoing individuals, by the same token. In any case, the genuine issue comes when loners don't get themselves and end up reasoning something is off-base with them. Albeit mistaken, this decision really appears to be legit, particularly when you take a gander at a portion of the current definition in regards to contemplation. I was stunned by how bad some of them were. Peruse on for probably the most disrupting ones (however don't feel excessively discouraged, we will bust those legends in this book).

- The Dictionary of Psychology states that introversion is, "… orientation inward toward the self. The introvert is preoccupied with his own thoughts, avoids social contact, and tends to turn away from reality."
- Webster's New Collegiate Dictionary describes introversion as, "… the state or tendency toward being wholly or predominantly concerned with and interested in one's own mental life."
- In what is perhaps the most negative definition of all, Webster's New World Thesaurus claims that the words 'brooder', 'self-observer', 'egoist', 'narcissist', 'solitary', 'lone wolf', and 'loner' are synonyms for 'introvert'.

Judging by those definitions, being a contemplative person doesn't seem like a lot of fun! Indeed, it seems like something terrible to be. This asks the accompanying questions:

- Why are introverts so different from extroverts?
- Is it possible for introverts to become extroverts, and
- Is there any reason that they should?

Action step

Before we characterize what self preoccupation is, pause for a minute to compose your own definition in the workbook.

(Section I. *Getting Introversion - 1. Your own meaning of introversion.*)

Introverts vs. Extroverts – The Genetic Factor

Whether we're thoughtful or outgoing is by all accounts generally controlled by our science, which implies that we can't transform it—it's a piece of what our identity is. All things considered, loners are fit for behaving like outgoing people as well as the other way around, yet just temporarily. This, obviously, requires an individual to get back to their regular state to re-energize their batteries.

What recognizes contemplative people from social butterflies is the manner in which they make and devour passionate energy. Outgoing individuals need a great deal of incitement from the rest of the world. Without it, they begin losing energy and start to feel exhausted, desolate, or tired. Loners need less outside incitement and time spent in friendly circumstances will generally exhaust their energy. This thusly drives them to pull out and invest energy alone to restore themselves.

It's pivotal for contemplative people to comprehend that being independent isn't as old as bashful. Despite the fact that there is some connection between's the two, they are two distinct things. Not all self observers are bashful. Then again, a few outgoing individuals are timid, which can be particularly disappointing. In the event that you're a modest outgoing person, you need to talk however you can't! We'll address timidity at more length later in this book.

The "Why" Behind Responses to Stimulus

There are really logical physiological motivations behind why outgoing people need more incitement: they're more delicate to the synapse dopamine than loners. Indeed, the prevailing synapses of the two gatherings are unique: contemplative people use acetylcholine as their essential synapse, while social butterflies depend on dopamine. Acetylcholine is made through feeling and thinking, and its essence expands center, upgrades memory, and cultivates a feeling of prosperity. One might say that loners auto-animate by investing energy thinking, noticing, or contemplating.

Extroverts, then again, need to make more dopamine, which frequently requires adrenaline. Expanding action and searching out incitement are both proficient ways of sloping up adrenaline. The requirement for dopamine and adrenaline is a significant justification for why outgoing people will quite often face greater challenges than loners. Hazard taking gives that additional incitement that social butterflies need. They are more award situated and will generally get exhausted when left alone for a really long time. Therefore, they will generally lose concentration and feel more awful than thoughtful people when under-stimulated.

In, The Introvert ADvantage, Martin Olsen Laney, Psy.D. composed the accompanying on how the utilization of various synapses can clarify contrasts among contemplative people and extroverts:

> *I think the link between which neurotransmitters travel what pathways and how they connect with different parts of the autonomic nervous center is the master key to unlocking the temperament puzzle. Whereas extroverts are linked with the dopamine adrenaline, energy-spending sympathetic nervous system, introverts are connected with the acetylcholine, energy conserving parasympathetic nervous system.*

Further tests demonstrate that self observers are more effortlessly invigorated than outgoing individuals. This affectability clarifies why, when placed in a loud or swarmed climate, loners wind up being overwhelmed, while outgoing individuals thrive.

In a 1967 test, Eysenck set lemon juice on the tongues of individuals who he recognized as thoughtful people and social butterflies. He needed to distinguish any intra-bunch contrasts in paces of salivation. As he expected, during this test, loners delivered more salivation than outgoing individuals, demonstrating a propensity for loners to be more stirred by tactile stimuli.

In another notable test, loners and social butterflies were approached to take part in a difficult word game. The game included learning through experimentation. Members were needed to wear earphones that transmitted commotion and were allowed to change the volume as they saw fit. All things considered, outgoing people changed the volume to 72 decibels, while loners pick a lower volume of 55 decibels. Curiously, the review uncovered that, under these conditions, the two outgoing people and loners were similarly animated and played equally well.

More shockingly, when social butterflies played the game at the commotion level chose by self observers, as well as the other way around, the two outgoing individuals and loners failed to meet expectations. Each gathering required altogether more endeavors prior to finishing the game. So, social butterflies were under-animated, and thoughtful people over-invigorated, which at last prompted inferior performances.

Most importantly self observers, are more effectively animated than outgoing individuals. We'll perform at our best under moderate tactile improvements. Then again, outgoing individuals should be presented to more incitement to have the option to thrive.

It is essential to take note of that, albeit the vast majority think introspection and extroversion are the main two choices, they really exist on inverse sides of a continuum. This implies it's feasible to be an ambivert, or rather, somebody who has parts of both contemplation and extroversion. So where might you put yourself on the continuum?

The story of Professor Little

The accompanying story of educator Little is a decent delineation of what contemplation is and why we should figure out how to deal with our energy effectively.

Brian Little was a previous Harvard University brain research instructor and beneficiary of the 3M Teaching Fellowship, quite possibly the most renowned award an instructor can get. His understudies cherished him and his talks regularly finished with overwhelming applauses. He would often sing or make jokes during the classes. He seems like an outgoing individual, isn't that right? All things considered, he wasn't! That couldn't possibly be more off-base. He was profoundly independent and would invest his free energy perusing and composing or scoring music in his home, which was situated in the Canadian woods.

One day, Professor Little visited the Royal Military College Saint-Jean on the Richelieu River to give a discourse to a gathering of military officials. His speech was so well-received that they invited him each year.

There was one major problem, though. When his discourse finished, they welcomed him to go along with them for lunch. It was a bad dream for

Professor Little. He had one more talk to convey in the early evening and required a few "personal" chance to re-energize his battery. Luckily, he thought of an extraordinary thought. He created an enthusiasm for transport plan and inquired as to whether he could take a stroll along the waterway to appreciate boats all things considered. You can envision his alleviation when this empowered him to effectively decay the lunch offer.

He kept on doing this every year and go for strolls along the stream to re-energize after his talks. At some point, be that as it may, his discourse was moved to an alternate area. He froze. How might he track down a calm spot to rest? He utilized the last card in his grasp, which was the bathroom. He blockaded himself in a washroom slow down to keep away from collaborations with others.

Does this sound recognizable to you?

Professor Little's story represents that, as self observers, we can go about as outgoing individuals for some time, yet will ultimately have to re-energize our batteries. Thus, on the off chance that you need to convey a discourse, do a Facebook Live, or go to systems administration occasions, you can do it. Simply ensure you plan time to re-energize your battery.

The Key Characteristics of Introverts

Now, we should view a few essential qualities shared by far most of self observers, who tend to:

- Spend time alone to replenish themselves
- Dislike small talk but enjoy deep conversation
- Prefer small groups
- Think before they speak
- Require an invitation before they speak
- Avoid speaking until they feel they have something important to say
- Listen more than they talk
- Talk a lot when the topic is something they're passionate about
- Choose depth over breadth (they would rather know a few people very well than know several people casually)
- Keep their enthusiasm and excitement for themselves and share only with people they know very well
- Prefer to know a lot about a small cluster of topics than know a little

bit about a wide range of topics
- Need alone time to think (rather than having to endure brainstorming sessions)
- Dislike interruptions
- Be uncomfortable with conflict, and
- Need a lot of preparation before addressing an audience and have difficulties speaking for long periods of time.

Debunking the Myths: What Introverts Are Not

There are numerous fantasies encompassing inner-directedness. In this part, I'd prefer to invest some energy exposing the most widely recognized ones.

Myth 1: Introverts need to be fixed

Fact: Introversion is anything but a psychological problem. In 2010, there was a proposition to remember self preoccupation for the Diagnostic and Statistical Manual of Mental Disorders, which is viewed as the Bible of emotional wellness analyze. Similarly as with anything, introspection can coincide with emotional wellness issues, yet the proposition was dismissed. Except if you're withdrawn to the point that it holds you back from working consistently, you don't have anything to stress about.

Myth 2: Introverts lack social skills

Fact: Social abilities can be mastered, and, except if particularly timid, contemplative people can speak with others similarly just as outgoing individuals. They will quite often be great audience members, which frequently gives them an edge over extroverts.

Myth 3: Introverts don't care about other people

Fact: Introverts are as inspired by individuals as any other person, and are regularly more keen on individuals than most. This is essential for why they will more often than not avoid casual banter. Loners would much prefer get to know individuals on a more profound level. As Laurie Helgoe, creator of Introvert Power clarified, *"We should clear one thing up*: Introverts don't despise casual conversation since we loathe individuals. We disdain casual banter since we disdain the obstruction it makes between individuals." Well-said!

Myth 4: Introverts don't like to talk

Fact: This might appear to be valid in large gatherings, however with regards to little social affairs and one-on-one discussions, thoughtful people can (and will!) jabber. This is particularly evident on the off chance that they know a ton about the current subject or feel firmly about it.

I may not talk much in social environments, yet in case I'm with a couple of companions it very well may be difficult to quiet me down! I've certainly needed to remind myself to talk less at specific focuses, and there have been a couple of times where I've had a companion illuminate me that I'm gabbing. It's consistently an astonishment to me and my first idea is, "Truly? I had no idea!"

However, just like the case with most loners, this all relies on how well I realize individuals I'm conversing with. When the gathering begins to surpass five or six individuals, I start to talk extensively less. One-on-one discussions are my beloved type of correspondence since they permit me to look into an individual. What are they enthusiastic about? What are their qualities? What are their interests? What are their fantasies? Et cetera. While I can't represent each contemplative person in the world, I can say that the larger part I've met get a kick out of discussions like that.

Introverts internalize, extroverts externalize

> *Extroverts often incorrectly assume that introverts are suffering. Introverts internalize problems; we like to take things inside and work on them there. Extroverts prefer to externalize and deal with problems interactively.*
>
> — LAURIE HELGOE, AUTHOR OF INTROVERT POWER.

Introverts like to disguise things. We like to thoroughly consider issues to them instead of examining them with others. We like to search inside to take care of our own concerns instead of offering our concerns to others to track down an answer. We are at our best when we can think alone peacefully. We don't do close to too when we're relied upon to conceptualize with a gathering and concoct good thoughts on the spot.

Similarly, we like to think before we talk, and have commonly a ton of hardships talking without notice. Then again, outgoing individuals talk first and afterward, refine their thinking as they talk. It isn't to say that single direction is better compared to the next, yet that self observers and social butterflies articulate their thoughts differently.

While now and again overthinking can be an issue for loners, we by and large are fine the manner in which we are and don't should be fixed.

Introversion doesn't equal shyness

Many individuals experience issues separating inner-directedness from shyness.
However, these states are not the equivalent, and it is significant that, as contemplative people, we separate the two.

Being a thoughtful person, it alludes to the manner in which we make and burn-through passionate energy. It doesn't imply that we need self-assurance or are reluctant to converse with individuals. Assuming that is the situation, it's a different issue, since individuals of all character types can, on occasion, battle with certainty and fear.

Many loners will really jabber during profound discussions, however observe casual conversation depleting. The inclination is we should talk just when we have something important to say, not on the grounds that it's expected of us. Constraining themselves to talk when they would rather not requires a significant exertion from them and will rapidly drain their energy. Different types of improvement that social butterflies frequently appreciate, like uproarious spots, splendid lights, swarms, or new circumstances will likewise deplete their energy.

As a loner myself, it took me some time to separate between my self preoccupation and bashfulness. As I acquired certainty in the course of recent years I found that I'm not an especially timid individual. I don't really feel timid in huge gatherings of individuals or while participating in gab, yet I actually abstain from talking when I don't have the energy for it. Certain circumstances require more energy than I have and it is that, rather than timidity, which holds me back from being the bigmouth I have in some cases wished I was. After some time, I've become dynamically more mindful of the tremendous contrasts among contemplation and shyness.

When I go to a party, I typically don't have a clue who I should converse with. There's not sufficient opportunity to get to know many individuals and I'm not enamored with easygoing discussions. I typically wind up having a one-on-one discussion with at least one or two individuals (this is the most ideal choice for me, if I'm conversing with intriguing individuals!) or meandering gracelessly from one gathering to another, depleted and uncertain of what to do. That, obviously, is the most dire outcome imaginable. Loners don't get invigorated through associating all by itself, however we can get siphoned up and surprisingly exceptional when discussions go to themes we're enthusiastic about.

I can't pressure sufficient that comprehend the distinction among introspection and bashfulness. At the point when individuals become familiar with this distinction, it offers them a chance to reconsider whether they're really timid and empowers them to

break liberated from culpability. Working on fearlessness is hard enough all alone, so don't make it significantly more troublesome by befuddling self preoccupation and modesty. Doing as such can prompt sat around idly attempting to change something that can't be changed, which will eventually end in discouragement.

It's not strange to feel tired in the wake of investing bunches of energy with individuals. You're not drained in light of the fact that you're bashful, need to get out additional, or need to become accustomed to conversing with individuals. You're recently contemplative, and there's nothing off about that.

It's alright in case you can't talk at a gathering without getting ready in advance. It's alright in case individuals around you seem like masters since they can convey smooth discourses suddenly. They may not be any more brilliant than you. There's nothing to stress over assuming you can't think unmistakably while in a huge gathering. I've seen that it's exceptionally difficult for me to concoct truly smart thoughts or think profoundly when I'm essential for a gathering. I do my best thinking in isolation. You don't have to feel awful in the event that you struggle with babble or on the other hand assuming you don't want to talk. Also assuming individuals think that you are exhausting or dull on the grounds that you don't talk a lot, that is OK, too.

I feel that loners will quite often appear to be modest in light of the fact that connecting with individuals is burdening for them. Therefore, they have less experience conversing with individuals than outgoing people do, and hence have a more extreme expectation to absorb information than outgoing people with regards to building social abilities. In addition, extroversion is the standard in numerous nations, despite the fact that self observers represent half of the total populace. Tragically, schools and workplaces aren't intended for self observers. Many thoughtful people spend their lives being informed that they should talk and mingle more, which regularly prompts culpability and sensations of low confidence that social butterflies are more averse to experience.

That said, be mindful so as not to take cover behind your introspection. Make certain to loosen up from your usual range of familiarity from time to time.

I comprehend that separating introspection from modesty can be interesting. Here's something I need you to pursue the following fourteen days: at whatever point you interface with individuals, set aside effort to see how you feel. For instance:

- Do you feel shy and awkward, or are you simply not in a talking mood?
- Are you feeling drained or timid?
- Do you feel more comfortable with one-on-one conversations, or do you feel awkward, timid, and shy regardless of how many people are involved in the discussion?

Try to distinguish the sentiments that surface during every one of your discussions. In the event that you persistently look at your sentiments and practices, it'll be a lot simpler to differentiate among modesty and introversion.

Action step

Using your workbook, complete the following exercise (Section I. *Understanding introversion):*

- Write down your relationship with introversion (ex: I feel ashamed, I feel guilty, I feel frustrated etc.).
- Differentiate introversion from shyness by asking yourself: Why aren't I talking? Then write whether your reasons are based on shyness (feeling scared and uncomfortable) or introversion (feeling too low on energy). For shyness write "S", for introversion write "I".
-

Write down your expectations regarding this book. Why did you buy this book and what do you want to get out of it? (e.g., improving my relationship with my partner, becoming better at networking, acceptation my introversion etc.)

2

OWNING YOUR INTROVERSION

Unfortunately for self observers, we experience a daily reality such that is fundamentally intended for social butterflies. Extroversion is the prevailing model of predictability and many self observers think that it is hard to fit in. Large numbers of us make a decent attempt to become outgoing people, just to wind up baffled and depleted. We're told we should take more, be more friendly, and show more drive. At times, we are even considered to be inflated, unapproachable, or exhausting!

Be that as it may, self preoccupation shouldn't be viewed as a weight. It's not something that must be fixed, nor is it anything to be embarrassed about. An incredible opposite, contemplation ought to really be embraced. As contemplative people, we have a ton to add to the world. As verified in the past section, it's assessed that around half individuals in this world are independent to changing degree. Who might have speculated? Extroversion is given such a lot of consideration and applause you'd think outgoing individuals represent most of the populace. But that's simply not true.

Introverts aren't feeble animals who need to buck up a behave like outgoing people to satisfy cultural guidelines. If, following huge number of long periods of development, contemplative people actually represent half of the populace, it is clear we play our part to play in the public arena. That is really significant, and we can't be overlooked. A long period of time of advancement can't be wrong.

In this segment, I'll urge you to accept your introspection and lose any culpability, disgrace or dissatisfaction you feel in regards to it. As a loner, you play a part to play, and that job doesn't include professing to be an outgoing individual. That would be pointless.

Action step

Before we get everything rolling, utilize the exercise manual to address the accompanying inquiries (Section II. *Possessing your contemplation - 1. Your greatest challenge):*

- What is my biggest challenge as an introvert?
- What could I do to overcome it?
- What is the one thing that would have the biggest positive impact on my life?

Why your assumptions on introversion matter more than you think

> *Begin challenging your own assumptions. Your assumptions are your windows on the world. Scrub them off every once in while, or the light won't come in.*
>
> — ALAN ALDA, ACTOR, SCREENWRITER AND AUTHOR.

We all have suppositions about existence. We anticipate that things should be a sure way, and we have explicit convictions on how we figure we ought to act. As a self observer, you hold numerous suspicions that you might know nothing about. These presumptions can keep you from accepting your introspection. An indication of a supposition that is the utilization of the expression "I ought to". At the point when you utilize that expression, you're probably expressing a suspicion. So why not require a couple of moments to think about every one of the suspicions identified with your introversion?

The assumptions you have in regards to your conduct can make pointless experiencing in your life. At the point when you accept you ought to act like a social butterfly, you'll regret yourself when you don't or can't support the conduct. You might have the option to carry on like a social butterfly on an intermittent premise, but

it isn't normal to act that way if, where it counts, you are a thoughtful person. It must be done on an impermanent premise, so you'll be hopeless in case you figure you should behave like a social butterfly continually.

The initial move towards tolerating your introspection is taking a gander at every one of the presumptions you hold with respect to it. As you do this, you'll understand that a considerable lot of your suspicions are in reality off-base. The following are a few instances of suppositions that you may hold.

- I'm boring if I'm not talking.
- Silence is awkward, so I should talk to avoid it.
- I don't enjoy parties, so something must be wrong with me.
- I shouldn't stay home on a Friday night.
- If I don't like talking to people because I'm shy.
- If I open my mouth, I'd better say something interesting.

You might think you have not many presumptions, yet you really have thousands in every part of our life. For instance, we should zero in on some particular suspicions you might have when you're at a party:

- I should continue listening to this person who's talking non-stop for ages because breaking off the conversation would be rude.
- Taking a break to go for a walk during a party is weird.
- I should talk more.
- It's normal to feel guilty for talking too little.
- I should enjoy the party.
- I should have more energy.
- I should stay until the end of the party.
- I should say something interesting.
- *Everyone else having a good time, so what's my problem?

*Remember that loners represent half of the populace, so you're only one of many individuals who loathes parties!

Action step

Use the exercise manual to record assumptions that straightforwardly impact the manner in which you experience your inner-directedness. (Segment I. *Claiming your inner-directedness - 2. Testing your assumptions)*

Accepting Yourself as You Are

> *Don't think of introversion as something that needs to be cured ... Spend your free time the way you like, not the way you think you're supposed to.*
>
> — SUSAN CAIN.

Do you apologize for being tall or short? What might be said about for taking care of business or a lady? On the off chance that you don't apologize for any of these things (and you shouldn't, you truly shouldn't), why would it be advisable for you to apologize for being a thoughtful person? Inner-directedness isn't something you can turn on and off freely. It's anything but a decision that you make. You want some alone an ideal opportunity to re-energize your energy, and that won't change. It's exactly how your cerebrum functions. Period.

Sure, you might have the option to carry on like an outgoing person for a couple of hours, however it doesn't change the way that you really want some 'alone' an ideal opportunity to re-energize your batteries. Forgetting to do that implies disregarding yourself and conflicting with your own nature.

You aren't lacking anything

> *...the most important thing to know about being an introvert is that there's nothing wrong with you. You're not broken because you're quiet. It's okay to stay home on a Friday night instead of going to a party. Being a loner is an entirely typical 'thing' to be.*
>
> — JENN GRANNEMAN, AUTHOR OF THE SECRETS LIVES OF INTROVERTS.

People regularly consider loners to be inadequate with regards to something. A few outgoing individuals say that we need, indeed, extroversion. They let us know we should talk more, go out additional, and live it up additional. But people who do this are simply projecting their extroverted nature onto us.

You don't have to profess to be outgoing to make up for your introspection, since you're not lacking anything. You don't should be restored. You're not insane, gaudy, or off-kilter. You don't have to turn into an outgoing individual. You simply need to comprehend and regard yourself for who you are.

You don't owe anyone social interactions

> *I don't hate people, I just feel better when they aren't around.*
>
> — CHARLES BUKOWSKI, POET.

We regularly accept that we want to collaborate with others. We "ought to" pick up the telephone when somebody calls, we "ought to" say something fascinating to stay away from quiets in discussion, or we "ought to" keep a discussion going.

Well, that is false. No one has the privilege to drive social communications upon you. No one is permitted to utilize your valuable time without your consent. You can go to a party without conversing with anybody in the event that you so decide. You can leave a discussion whenever by saying something like, "It was great conversing with you, yet I must get rolling. I'll converse with you later".

Nobody is qualified for your time. It's not possible for anyone to squander your restricted energy except if you permit them to. Consider it along these lines: when an outgoing individual discussions to you, *they fell great since they need to connect with individuals to re-energize themselves*. It could be said, you fill a need for them. However that still

doesn't mean you should keep the discussion going just to be courteous. It's draining the energy out of you, and anyone who anticipates that you should bear that interminably is really narrow minded. Would you compel a social butterfly to remain at home and read books since that is what invigorates you? Obviously not.

Remember, you don't owe anyone social connection! Since cooperating with individuals drains your energy, be specific with regards to who you converse with and for how long.

You don't have to talk

> *A wise man once said nothing.*
>
> — PROVERB.

What assuming I let you know that you don't need to talk? Talking more doesn't make you a superior person. I used to battle with this thought. I generally felt like I expected to say something. I accepted that I should have been talking. All things considered, I felt something was off-base with me on the off chance that I remained quiet.

A couple of months prior, I was at a party with my work associates, when abruptly, something horrendous occurred: A respite in the overall discussion. Goodness! Please, somebody say something, anything! I was having a different one-on-one discussion with somebody at that point, and, when clearly I wasn't joining the gathering discussion, somebody requested that I say something. I answered, "I have nothing to say and, frankly, I like the quiet." As you can see, contemplation is done something I'm embarrassed about. I had the option to say unhesitatingly and without culpability, that I had nothing to say. I wouldn't have had the option to do that a couple of years prior. Shockingly, many individuals fear quiet. Perhaps, they're worried about the possibility that that they aren't adequately fascinating. Or then again perhaps, they like to zero in on the outer world to abstain from glimpsing inside. In numerous ways, quietness can be extremely incredible, and furthermore very enjoyable.

You don't need to apologize for the way you feel

Remember that individuals can contend with what you say, however they can't contend with how you feel. How you feel is the manner by which you feel. That is it. Assuming you feel tired and need to return home or enjoy some time off, do that. Despite what individuals say, you're answerable for your energy and how you oversee it.

You don't need to feel ashamed or guilty

> *What a commentary on our civilization, when being alone is considered suspect; when one has to apologize for it, make excuses, hide the fact that one practices it like a secret vice!*
>
> — ANNE MORROW LINDBERGH, AUTHOR.

It's not difficult to feel embarrassed or remorseful in light of the fact that you don't talk however much you'd like or loath gatherings in the manner you "ought to". You might fault yourself for not having sufficient energy or accepting you ought to have a greater amount of it. You might even dislike yourself for being not able to take part in casual discussion or be the focal point of consideration. I once felt the equivalent way.

The thing is, there's nothing off about the manner in which you act, nor is there anything amiss with the manner in which outgoing individuals act. Your sentiments and practices aren't abnormal or odd. Don't "ought to" yourself. Relinquish your coerce and do what you genuinely need to do.

You don't need to be jealous of extroverts

This is a troublesome one since I presume many loners covertly wish they were outgoing people. Perhaps you have that impression, as well. You might begrudge social butterflies for their capacity to interface with such ease with others. You begin envisioning the amount more famous you'd be in the event that you were an outgoing individual. You may occasion disdain them somewhat. I positively did. In this case, you may make a decent attempt to work on yourself to turn out to be seriously fascinating (be it through considering, going to the exercise center, or sharpening another ability), just to wind up unseen and with nothing to say.

Half a month prior, I went over one remark I saw as difficult to neglect. The remark expressed that self observers couldn't be cheerful, as they all begrudged social butterflies. Obviously, I thought it was BS.

We might accept that social butterflies are cheerful constantly, yet that is not the situation. Social butterflies depend more on outer components (like individuals) to re-energize themselves. At times, this prompts depending on others and others' endorsement for their own satisfaction. They might think that it is hard to invest energy without help from anyone else and may get desolate without any problem. Loners, then again, are frequently cheerful by themselves.

It's additionally imperative to recall that being a self observer doesn't mean you can't cooperate with others or be an incredible conversationalist. Those things are absolutely conceivable, however you'd must be somewhat more key by they way you deal with your time and re-energize yourself.

It's worth focusing on here, that one of the principle reasons thoughtful people might be troubled is an overall absence of comprehension. We make a decent attempt to be somebody else. We take a gander at ourselves from a perspective that is one-sided towards extraversion, and afterward judge ourselves dependent on that imperfect worldview. All in all, our fundamental suppositions aren't right. As I said previously, this makes wrong assumptions and prompts superfluous suffering.

Action step

Answer the accompanying inquiries utilizing the exercise manual (Section II. *Possessing your self preoccupation - 3. Tolerating your introversion)*

- How well do you own your introversion? Write down one negative feeling you associate with it (e.g.: feeling guilty for not talking enough, feeling tired, etc.)
- Name thing you could do or one belief you could adopt that would help you let go of that negative feeling?
- What positive feelings and emotions do you associate with your introversion? Try to write down as many as possible. (E.G. enjoying spending time at home, taking pleasure in reading a new book etc.)

OPTIMIZING YOUR INTROVERSION

Are you by and large empowered for the duration of the day, or do you feel depleted the greater part of the time?

In this segment, we'll talk about how you can upgrade your day to suit your thoughtful character. The principal thing I'd like you to do is imagine your optimal day. What might it resemble? What might you do? How might you spend your time?

As it stands, you might need to invest energy connecting with heaps of individuals at wOr on the other handk in spite of leaning toward little gatherings. Or, you may have an accomplice who habitually has companions over, making it hard to unwind alone.

For the occasion, disregard your life as it is presently. Simply imagine what your ideal day would look like.

Action step

Use the exercise manual to writ down what your ideal day would comprise of. (Segment III. *Upgrading your inner-directedness - 1. Planning your ideal day)*

- Imagine you're living the perfect life as an introvert. What does your typical day look like? What are you doing? Who are you spending your time with? How much time do you spend alone?
- What's preventing you from living like this? What's holding you back?
- What's the one thing you could do today to move you closer to the vision you have for yourself?
- Add one more thing you could do

Managing your energy - the key to a happy life

> *I'm very picky with whom I give my energy to. I prefer to reserve my time, intensity and spirit exclusively to those who reflect sincerity.*
>
> — DAU VOIRE,
> AUTHOR.

Have you at any point remained whatsoever party for a really long time just to leave feeling completely depleted? As loners, dealing with our energy is by a long shot probably our greatest test. Without satisfactory energy, we become unfit to work appropriately and eventually daydream. We become surly, worried, and miserable. A few of us even beginning having an embarrassed or liable outlook on our contemplative nature.

As you can see, figuring out how to utilize your energy carefully is critical. You shouldn't permit individuals or circumstances to exhaust your energy. It's your obligation to control these things. Your companions may say that you should go to a party since "it will be enjoyable" or pressure you to remain longer than you'd like. This is presumably benevolent, yet the reality stays that you are the one in particular who knows how you feel and what you need to do. I don't care for it when somebody lets me know what I ought to do dependent on what they need to do. I have an inclination that not a single one of us partake in that very much.

Telling a loner to remain at a party when they need to return home and re-energize resembles advising an outgoing individual to return home and read when they need to mingle and expand their energy. "Come on man, you're so exhausting! Return home and read a book!". It sounds pretty absurd when you put the situation reversed, doesn't it?

Finding your sweet spot

> *People empty me. I have to get away to refill.*
>
> — C. BUKOWSKI,
> AUTHOR.

As a self observer, you have restricted energy for mingling. The more you know yourself and comprehend your limits, the more you'll have the option to try not to feel depleted by the day's end. Track down your perfect balance, regardless of whether you're separated from everyone else or with people.

When you're by yourself

Introverts wouldn't fret remaining at home for a fun time. Contingent upon your degree of contemplation, remaining in for a day, end of the week, or significantly longer probably won't trouble you. Nonetheless, investing an excessive amount of energy alone can make it harder to associate on even the most fundamental levels.

Here's an inquiry to pose to yourself: How long would i be able to remain at home prior to going out and dealing with essential connections turns into a difficulty? Preferably, you need to try not to remain at home beyond this point. Keeping that in mind, it's great to get out consistently, regardless of whether not for the communicated motivation behind socializing.

Start seeing how you feel when you remain at home for a really long time, and start going out for something other than work. Here and there, being all alone for a really long time can become overpowering. Indeed, even thoughtful people need to mingle. In any case, we hazard harping on bad musings, feeling desolate, or getting hung up on something that is disturbing us.

When you're with others

How much time would you be able to spend at a get-together prior to running out of energy? For my purposes, it's several hours. After that point, I begin feeling equivalent amounts of exhausted and exhausting. I quit having fun. That is an indication that it's the ideal opportunity for me to leave! As far as you might be concerned, it could be two hours also, however it could effectively be pretty much. Obviously, it will likewise rely upon the circumstance and how much energy you start with. The following are a few factors that might affect how quick your energy is depleted:

- The loudness of the venue
- How crowded it is
- How interactive you're expected to be
- How formal the event is

- How many people you know
- How familiar you are with the venue
- Whether you can partake in activities besides talking

It's significant that you figure out how to screen your energy so you can more readily design your day. When you know your perfect balance, things will become simpler. Afterward, we'll examine how to manage parties as an introvert.

The importance of maintaining your space

As introverts, simply being around people can drain your energy, even when we aren't required to talk. You've likely been in circumstances where you're distant from everyone else in a room having a good time—until someone shows us. This could occur at the exercise center, in the library, or at a bistro, to give some examples models. In any of these circumstances, what occurred straightaway? How could it cause you to feel? On the off chance that you're in any way similar to me, you most likely felt somewhat irritated, restless, or depleted. I can't represent outgoing individuals, yet my speculation would be that this wouldn't be no joking matter for them. They may really get energized and initiate a discussion with the newcomer.

I disdain having individuals around when I'm attempting to appreciate something alone. While doing as such, I only occasionally welcome anybody to accompany me, and assuming I do, they need to be an amazingly dear companion. I attempt to try not to be with others when I need to partake in a space all alone. In that circumstance, companions of companions or colleagues would be the most noticeably awful individuals to be near, as I'd must choose the option to have some way of discussion with them.

Have you at any point made arrangements to get along with a companion possibly to have them inquire as to whether another person can go along? How could it feel? Chances are, you were anticipating having a profound discussion with your companion and felt it was destroyed by adding an in addition to one. I can thoroughly identify with that.

Also, when you are coming up short on energy, note that actual contact with individuals, even our accomplice or our relatives, might be overpowering. Sometimes, you may not need anyone close you.

Action step

Use the exercise manual to advance your degree of energy. (Segment III. *Enhancing your contemplation - 2. Dealing with your energy/3. Distinguishing your sweet spot)*

2. Managing your energy:

- What could you do to better manage your energy?
- What is the one thing that would have the biggest positive impact on your energy level?

3. Identifying your sweet spot:

Based on your own insight, how long would you be able to spend at a get-together prior to wanting to leave or enjoy some time off to re-energize your battery?

Optimizing Your Life

As a thoughtful person, you're probably going to deal with issues in different parts of your life. In this segment, I'd prefer to give you a few hints to enhance your life. I'll zero in on 3 distinct regions: your public activity, vocation, and relationships.

Your social life

> *Introverts crave meaning so party chitchat feels like sandpaper to our psyche.*
>
> — DIANE CAMERON.

As contemplative people, we regularly have an affection disdain relationship with get-togethers. A piece of us needs to go, yet we can't quit thinking, "Am

I going to partake in the party?" In the end, we regularly end up remaining at home. There's nothing bad about remaining at home, obviously, and parties aren't a need of life. All things considered, we as a whole need or need to go out to make companions or organization. I will examine how we can overhaul our public activities to make them more "self observer friendly".

Dealing with parties

Parties can be fun, yet they can likewise be a bad dream for loners assuming we don't deal with them appropriately. Remaining for a really long time can leave us totally depleted and wishing we hadn't come. But it doesn't have to be that way. Adapting to parties the thoughtful person way will make your life more straightforward and more enjoyable.

Deciding whether you should go

First of all, you want to choose if you really need to go to the occasion or party. In her book The Introvert Power, Laurie A. Helgoe gives the accompanying tips on concluding whether you ought to go.

- **How big is the party?** Usually, the bigger the party is, the more tiring it will be.
- **What is the setting?** Is it an indoor or outdoor event? Is there a lot of space or will it be crowded? How loud will it be? A beach party, for instance, will make it easier for you to take a break, go for walk, or leave when you're ready. On the other hand, an indoor party in a confined environment could quickly become overwhelming.
- **Do I know the people who will be attending?** If you know most of the people there, you'll feel more at ease. It goes without saying that not knowing anyone will likely be uncomfortable.
- **Are there any activities I can partake in that don't involve talking?** You'll typically feel more comfortable when you can do something besides talk. It makes interactions with other people much smoother. If all you can do is stand and talk, however (think cocktail parties), it'll be much more challenging.
- **Do I really want to go?** Based on your previous answers, ask yourself this: "On a scale of 1 to 10, how excited am I about this party?" In other words, will I regret not having gone? Some introverts fear that they may be missing out. So, keep that in mind when

you make your decision.

Learning to say "no"

There's an amazingly basic and profoundly compelling method for dealing with parties you're uncertain about (or don't have any desire to go to): Just don't go! That will tackle large numbers of your concerns. While it sounds adequately simple, many individuals battle to decrease solicitations and going to parties when they don't need to.

The primary thing to comprehend is that gatherings are definitely not an unquestionable requirement. No one has the privilege to compel you to join in. It frequently appears like gatherings are the best way to have a great time. I don't be aware of you, be that as it may, as far as I might be concerned, having some espresso with a couple of dear companions can be more fulfilling than going to a party. The equivalent goes for perusing a decent book. Parties are misrepresented, and I speculate that many individuals (generally self observers) loath them by any means. They simply claim to. I don't know whether or not you appreciate parties, yet assuming you don't, I would encourage you to quit claiming to. The greater part of us invest an excessive amount of energy imagining or attempting to fit in. We claim to be content, we profess to like our positions, we imagine our relationship is extraordinary, thus on.

Whatever you decide to do with your time is fine as long as it's credible. There's no compelling reason to counterfeit anything.

How to say "no"

So, you've chosen to decay your companion's encouragement to savor brews an uproarious Irish bar on Friday night. Presently, you don't know how to tell them. Your companion believes you're insane and is now letting you know how much fun it will be. "You will adore it," he says. I keep thinking about whether he would acknowledge your encouragement to come over and read books peacefully. He would simply adore that, right?

Think of saying no as an indication of self confidence. You ought to likewise remember that, assuming you need outgoing individuals to quit dealing with you like a social butterfly, you need to accept your introspection. On the off chance that you continually apologize for skipping things you would have rather not go to regardless, how might you anticipate that extroverts should change their conduct towards you? They will not have the option to comprehend your requirement for isolation assuming you convey conflicting messages. The following are four hints to assist you with saying no:

1. Stop apologizing: You don't need to apologize for wanting to spend your time in a way that will maximize your happiness! You don't try to keep extroverts from expressing their extroversion. You don't attempt to prevent them from celebrating the entire evening assuming that is the thing that they need to. It's their life, correct? In this way, don't allow others to do that to you. There's no compelling reason to say, "I'd prefer to go, however…." If you continue to say that, odds are individuals will keep on welcoming you, which probably won't be what you need.
2. Own your introspection: Instead of saying that you "want" to rest, state unmistakably it's what you need. "I'm anticipating perusing an extraordinary book around evening time," or "I need some an ideal opportunity to myself," or "I'm amped up for remaining in and unwinding." This will preferred pass on your plan over, "I want to rest."
3. Be straightforward: Say things as they are and embrace your contemplation. The more your regard yourself and acknowledge your contemplation, the more your companions will acknowledge it, as well. Keep in mind, many individuals don't get contemplation. Your genuine companions will be more steady once they get what your requirements are. They'll uphold your decision to remain at home, yet will likewise assist you with saving your energy during parties, which we'll cover later on. You can say something like, "You know, I'm not enthusiastic about parties. I had a debilitating week and I'm anticipating remaining at home and perusing an extraordinary book."
4. Offer other options (discretionary): Sometimes you need to get up with your companions, however not in that packed Irish bar on Friday night. Assuming that is the situation, you can just offer another choice. You could say, "I've had a debilitating week and I will re-energize my batteries by perusing an incredible book this evening. But I really want to catch up with you, so let's have a coffee this Sunday." That's a decent method for showing that you would like to see your companions, yet not at an uproarious, overpowering scene. You might even specify that you'll have further discussions. This will enjoy the benefit of assisting them with understanding the worth of your friendship.

Additional tip: It's hard to assert yourself in a society where extroversion appears to be the norm. It's considerably harder when many individuals view introspection as something that requires "fixing". Obviously, standing up for yourself takes some preparation. Try not to stop for a second to rehearse with a companion or all alone. For example, you could make a few expressions that permit you to courteously decrease occasions you're not inspired by. Pick reactions that impact you and practice them until you feel adequately sure to utilize them in a genuine discussion. Look at the accompanying examples:

- Thanks, but I really prefer small gatherings.
- Thanks, but I'm focusing on *insert project or goal here* and can't deal with distractions at the moment.
- Thanks, but I don't really go to parties, I prefer intimate gatherings with just a few friends.

Try moving yourself to be straightforward while staying amiable and see what happens.

You may likewise need to allude to the rundown of insistences toward the finish of this book. Go ahead and utilize the ones that impact you on consistent schedule or make your own.

Dealing with parties the introvert way

Let's say you acknowledge the party greeting, ideally in light of the fact that you genuinely need to

go, however start re-thinking yourself. "Am I truly going to partake in the party? Will I lament not having remained at home?" When you go to a party, there's in every case some degree of vulnerability. In some cases, I've gone to a party without assumptions and lived it up. Different occasions, I've been really energized uniquely to wind up exhausted and disillusioned. Luckily, as contemplative people, there are numerous things we can do to expand our odds of living it up. Consider the accompanying tactics:

Arriving early: Assuming it's good with the host, showing up sooner than expected to a party permits you to find out about the climate and begin cooperating with a more modest pool of individuals. It very well might be simpler to have one-on-one discussions or talk with a little gathering before everybody shows up. The scene will be calmer and less crowded.

Leaving right on time: As contemplative people, we can indeed invest a limited amount a lot of energy in an excessively animating climate. There's literally nothing amiss with leaving early. Of late, I will quite often show up after the expected time and leave early, seldom remaining in excess of a few hours. The justification behind that? Following two or three hours, I loath myself any longer, so I simply leave. Also you ought to, as well! There's not a good excuse to remain after you quit having a great time. At the point when individuals ask me for what reason I'm so late I answer that I had some work to do (like composing this book). With regards to leaving, ensure you have your departure plan prepared before you go.

Bringing an outgoing companion: Remember, social butterflies are not the foe. Going to a party with an outgoing companion is an incredible method for assisting you with loosening things up and connect with a greater number of individuals than you would all alone. There are many individuals that I couldn't have ever met if not for my outgoing companions. Your companion will do a large portion of the talking, permitting you to safeguard your valuable energy.

Another advantage is that they'll probably praise you, which is more believable than if you somehow happened to say them yourself. That might prove to be useful, particularly if your'e searching for an accomplice. The majority of us don't care for talking ourselves up, so it's great to have a "PR" individual as your companion. I'm extremely appreciative for my outgoing companions. I trust you're appreciative for yours, too!

Briefing your outgoing friend(s) on your introspection: The more your companions comprehend your inner-directedness, the better they'll have the option to support

you. You need to have some time off from the party and take a walk? Don't sweat it, your companions will comprehend. You need to leave early? That is OK. In spite of the fact that they might need you to remain, your companions will understand.

Taking customary breaks: Don't spare a moment to enjoy incessant reprieves. This may mean taking a walk or going to the washroom. You could even ask the individual you're conversing with assuming the person in question needs to take a stroll with you.

For some explanation, we will more often than not hold convictions that keep us from acting unreservedly during get-togethers. However truly, you can go back and forth however you see fit, can leave a discussion whenever, you can take a thirty-minute walk, or you can go through fifteen minutes in the washroom (yet ensure you're not making a line!). You can do whatever you really want or need to do. Begin taking a gander at your own suppositions. You'll most likely observe that you're forcing counterfeit cutoff points on your conduct because of social molding. Consider breaking them!

Spotting different loners in the room: You probably will need to "target" different loners, as they may be more straightforward to approach. You'll most likely think that they are perched without anyone else or remaining toward the side of the room. Have a go at starting up a discussion with them and see where it goes. They may be more straightforward to converse with. Despite the fact that, being loners, don't be amazed or baffled assuming they say, "I'm glad all alone for the occasion." (Especially in case they've perused this book.)

Having out in an essential spot: You may decide to remain in a space where it'll be more straightforward for you to have one-on-one or little gathering discussions. You could remain in a corner, close to the kitchen, or in a passage, for example. Be watching out for regions that are calmer and less swarmed than others.

Volunteering: This is an incredible way for contemplative people to appreciate social cooperations without concocting something to discuss. You'll keep away from those off-kilter minutes where you don't have the foggiest idea who to converse with for sure to say. You will not need to nurture a beverage the entire evening or check your telephone continually to have something to do (I frequently do this!). You could, for example, be helping in the kitchen or taking pictures. It's by and large more straightforward for us to make associations when we're engaged with an action, like playing sports or cooking. Since we don't really need to move toward individuals and concoct a comment, the discussion streams more naturally.

Focusing on others to neglect ourselves: Switching your concentration from yourself to others can be a powerful method for decreasing your nervousness. You could, for instance, choose to go to a party with the target of gaining some new useful knowledge. You could even imagine a couple of inquiries you'd prefer to pose to somebody in advance. Utilizing this method, you'll be more centered around what you need to realize than you will be on your anxiety.

Setting explicit objectives: You can take a stab at laying out small objectives.

Your objective could be to move toward one gathering of individuals. When you achieve that small objective, you can return home glad. All that happens thereafter is simply what tops off an already good thing. In many cases, you might wind up moving toward a bigger number of individuals than you anticipate. The minuscule objective methodology can work for all aspects of your life. One of my minuscule objectives is to compose somewhere around 500 words each day, yet today I've as of now finished more than 2,000. The fact is, whatever you do can accelerate to great effect.

Escaping from a discussion: I used to remain in discussions for quite a long time since I incorrectly accepted it was inconsiderate to leave them. Bu here's reality: You don't owe anyone any cooperation, and it's not possible for anyone to deplete your energy or burn through your time without your assent. Presently, I basically say, "It was great talking with you. I'll converse with you later." Or, "My companion is hanging tight for me, it was great talking with you. I'll converse with you later." Try it for yourself the following time you feel caught in a discussion you feel has continued for too long.

Action step

Use the exercise manual (Section III. *Streamlining your self preoccupation - 4a. Streamlining your social life)*

- Regarding introversion, what are your biggest struggles in that area?
- What is one small thing you could do to improve your current situation in that area?

Your career

> *A good rule of thumb is that any environment that consistently leaves you feeling bad about who you are is the wrong environment.*
>
> — LAURIE HELGOE.

Do you feel completely depleted toward the finish of every day? On the off chance that you're working some unacceptable work or are in some unacceptable climate, you can undoubtedly feel overpowered. Perhaps you need to settle on telephone decisions for work and you disdain it. Or then again maybe meetings to generate new ideas and unlimited gatherings are depleting all your energy. Take some time to think of the things that, if you could do less of then, would make work more enjoyable.

Using our present models, this could mean settling on less telephone decisions or having a lower number of gatherings. After you've thought about a couple of things, record them. Also, ponder things that would make work simpler if you would accomplish a greater amount of them. This could be focusing on messages over calls. Record these things, too.

Unfortunately, the present common workplace isn't self observer agreeable. Open space is one of the most exceedingly terrible things for self observers. We would prefer to have more private space and calm chance to zero in on our work. The following are a few hints to assist you with upgrading your current circumstance and further develop your work fulfillment. Remember that this rundown is a long way from comprehensive. Everybody is unique, so I urge you to think of some particular and individual methodologies that work for you.

- Have lunch alone to give yourself some "me" time.
- Use your break to go for a walk.
- Look for empty conference rooms and use them to work without interruption.
- Arrive early or stay late to carve out some time alone.
- Wear headphones to prevent people from interrupting you.
- Negotiate working from home, even if it's just one afternoon per week. It will allow you to recharge your batteries. Make sure you stay useful, as that will place you in a superior situation to arrange investing more energy working from home.
- Ask your boss if you can send in ideas before or after a meeting. This will show that you're motivated and present even if you can't voice your opinions during meetings. Better still, you'll have more time after the meeting to put your ideas on paper.
- Tell your colleagues that you're working on minimizing interruptions throughout the day and ask them what they need from you. Request this from your most diverting colleagues.
- Let your boss and co-workers know that you'd like time to settle in in

the morning before talking to anyone.

- Clearly state that you'd prefer to communicate via email rather than by phone.
- Skip meetings whenever you can.
- Try setting office hours so as to create blocks of uninterrupted work time.

How to assert yourself at work

Because our inner-directedness is normal to us, we anticipate that those around we should think as we do, or essentially get us. In any case, loners and outgoing people think and act in an unexpected way. Your chief and associates don't really see you the manner in which you'd anticipate that they should. They may not understand the amount you're contributing. It is possible that you talk little since you don't understand the amount you know. Or on the other hand maybe you don't care for sharing your contemplations since it draws consideration. Individuals will not really get on things like this.

Most thoughtful people struggle shouting out and placing themselves at the center of attention. Individuals probably won't comprehend that you want time to think alone prior to talking, or that not speaking up during a gathering doesn't mean you're not able to contribute.

Check out the tips beneath to perceive how you can make your quality known.

1. Multiply one-on-one discussions: You probably won't have the option to contribute a lot during gatherings yet, as a self observer, you're for the most part great at talking to

individuals one-on-one. By setting out more open doors for one-on-one discussions, you can assemble further associations with your partners. You could, for example, welcome one of them to lunch. On the other hand, you could show up sooner than expected or remain late occasionally to initiate discussions with a portion of your colleagues previously (or after) everybody is in the workplace.

2. Offer your assistance: Volunteer for things that you have an interest in. Possibly you can compose a bulletin or offer a few articles with your associates. Or on the other hand you could propose some valuable assets. As contemplative people, we probably won't prefer to blow our own horns, however we commonly prefer to help. In view of what you know in regards to your associates or chief, how could you deal with help them? How might you assist them with accomplishing their own goals?

3. Focus on composed correspondence: Offer to share your musings and thoughts after a gathering. It will give you an opportunity to think and write your musings down while showing your longing to contribute.

4. Ask for help: Introverts might be hesitant to request help and should do everything all alone. Try not to surrender to this inclination. Requesting help is an extraordinary method for interfacing with your partners and cause them to feel appreciated. Many individuals like helping other people, so it's a shared benefit situation.

5. Keep your manager modern: You presumably don't speak with your supervisor as frequently as your outgoing colleagues do. You can make up for this by consistently telling your supervisor what you're up to.

Changing Careers

If you disdain your occupation since it doesn't permit you to flourish as a thoughtful person, it very well may be an ideal opportunity to think about tracking down another one. You probably won't have the option to change your work immediately. In any case, you want to ask yourself the accompanying inquiry: "Would I like to use the remainder of my life doing what I'm presently doing?" If not, why not plan for your future career?

Taking chance to plan your ideal day will assist you with picking a lifelong that suits you. You should ask yourself the accompanying questions:

- What are my strengths?
- What job would allow me to leverage these strengths?
- Do I want to spend most of my time alone, in one-on-one conversations, or conversing in small groups?
- How much of my time do I want to dedicate to these activities? *If you have no clue what you'd like to do in regard to a career, check out the paragraph on finding your passion in the section V, Transcending your introversion)*

Dealing with Networking Events

Networking occasions might be the last thing you need to join in. However, they're likely not quite as terrible as you might suspect. As opposed to mainstream thinking, there's no compelling reason to converse with everyone in the room or appropriate business cards by the dozen. Indeed, the individuals who do this for the most part end up with helpless outcomes. Remember that the tips referenced for parties function admirably for systems administration occasions also. Peruse on for nine hints on taking care of systems administration events:

1. Go profound: As a self observer, you probably want profound, significant discussions. I'm not sure why you ought to overlook that hankering when going to systems administration occasions. Put forward a little objective of building two or three significant collaborations rather than attempting to trade business cards with everybody in the room.

2. Set a reasonable objective: Before you go to a systems administration occasion, ensure you have a particular objective set. Ask yourself this: *What precisely am I attempting to accomplish here? For example*, your objective could be to make two significant associations. Having a reasonable objective that you're certain you can accomplish will assist with letting some free from the tension. Ensure, your objective isn't too huge. You can generally move toward a greater number of individuals than you set off to, yet that ought to be optional.

3. Decide how long you'll remain: Decide ahead of time how long you intend to spend at the occasion. It very well may be just twenty to thirty minutes. In the event that you wish to remain longer, go ahead and do as such, yet don't come down on yourself.

4. Prepare well: As contemplative people, we might battle to respond to inquiries on the spot or concoct great inquiries to pose. Subsequently, it's ideal to set up your inquiries early and practice replies to questions you might get. Ensure the inquiries you pose are open-finished. It's ideal to keep away from yes or no questions.

5. Create a straightforward short presentation: Put together a basic presentation you can utilize when you meet somebody interestingly. Attempt to see this brief presentation as your systems administration presentation. At the point when you present yourself, ensure you notice how you help individuals rather than zeroing in exclusively on what you do. What value do you offer and what problem(s) do you solve? Then, you want to state who precisely you'd like to connect with. View at your pitch as a secret whose goal is to urge individuals to pose inquiries that permit you to give more insights regarding what you do. Kathy McAfee from www.americasmarketingmotivator.com gives the following example[2]: "My name is , I'm a separation and family lawyer legal advisor. I assist individuals

with exploring through perhaps the most troublesome occasions in their life or "I assist individuals with settling on more astute decisions so they can proceed to have a glad life". Then, you can add, "I'm looking to connect with ".

6. Take breaks: You don't need to go to every one of the studios or remain for the entire occasion without a reprieve. Take however many breaks as you want, and do it without shame!

7. The 80/20 guideline: The 80/20 standard expresses that a fifth of our endeavors bring about the vast majority of our outcomes. The equivalent goes for systems administration occasions. Among the systems administration occasions that you think about joining in, some will offer a greater number of chances than others. As a thoughtful person, why not center around the 20% that are probably going to produce positive outcomes and skirt the rest?

8. Bring an outgoing companion: We examined this according to gatherings, and it has a comparable application here. Your outgoing companion will assist you with cooperating with more individuals and will remove the edge from things.

9. Follow-up: Make sure you circle back to individuals you connect with. Consider interfacing with them via online media stages and send them a special email dependent on what you examined at the event.

Networking the introvert way

Okay, so we've discussed organizing occasions, however who says you need to go

to them, at any rate? It's fine assuming that you decide to, however in case you would rather not, it's not the apocalypse. They aren't a need. There are alternate ways of systems administration that aren't close to as unpleasant and debilitating as conventional systems administration occasions. How about we examine some of them now.

Networking online

In this cutting edge age, we're adequately lucky to approach this thing called "The Internet". LinkedIn would be a decent spot to begin, yet you can observe numerous different locales or discussions identified with your industry that you can use for systems administration. You'll likewise track down huge loads of gatherings on Facebook. For example, I'm essential for a gathering of journalists on Facebook. I don't need to go to any occasions or even converse with anybody eye to eye to make asThusciations. The prospects are unending. So, assuming that you disdain organizing occasions, consider zeroing in just on a couple of occasions, or dispensing with them out and out. Zero in on your internet organizing instead.

Leveraging your personal network

You as of now have an individual organization, and every individual in your organization has their very own organization. Why not influence these networks?

For instance, one of your associates could acquaint you with somebody from an alternate industry that you'd prefer to look further into. You could then have an espresso with that person.

This would be a lot simpler than going to a systems administration occasion and trusting you'll get something out of it.

Action step

Use the exercise manual (Section III. *Improving your introspection - 4b. Improving your career)*

- Regarding introversion, what are your biggest struggles in this area?
- What is one small thing you could do to improve your current situation in that area?

Relationships

> *At every party, there are two kinds of people - those who want to go home and those who don't. The trouble is, they are usually married to each other.*

— ANN LANDERS, FAMOUS ADVICE COLUMNIST.

Is your accomplice a social butterfly? Do you have outgoing children? To guarantee satisfying connections, it's fundamental that outgoing individuals comprehend self observers' requirements (and bad habit versa).

Being in a relationship with an extrovert

If you're presently involved with a social butterfly, odds are the person in question consistently needs to welcome companions over and likes to go out on the ends of the week. This might even be a disputed matter between you. You wish you could possess more energy for you and didn't need to go through such countless ends of the week with companions or exploring through parties. Then again, your accomplice feels you're far off or introverted. The person might even be anxious about the possibility that that you don't adore them when you say you want alone time.

Below are a few hints that might assist you work on your relationship with your parter.

1. Make sure your accomplice gets what inner-directedness is and what it suggests: As an outgoing individual, your accomplice can't encounter inner-directedness. Thusly, the individual in question may not comprehend the reason why you really want to invest energy alone to re-energize your battery. It's fundamental that your accomplice comprehend your needs before you attempt to make changes in your relationship.

You could recommend the individual in question read a few books on self preoccupation (like this one, for example). The most ideal method for empowering your accomplice to more deeply study contemplation is to find out about extroversion yourself. Since let's be honest, you don't have the foggiest idea how it feels to be an outgoing person, by the same token. Ensure you invest some energy perusing a few articles or books on extroversion. Furthermore, ask your accomplice what challenges the individual in question experiences as a social butterfly. Recollect that the two outgoing people and self observers have difficulties. This common arrangement will roll out future improvements (and your coexistences) easier.

2. Express your necessities: Share your requirements with your accomplice.

Perhaps you wish you could have more opportunity to yourself, or additional time with simply you two, rather than being with companions constantly. Possibly you wish you could unwind on Friday night as opposed to going out with companions. Simply express your requirements and notice how your accomplice would profit from meeting them (for example, it may mean you're more accessible or are in a superior mood).

3. Listen to your accomplice's necessities, as well: Ask your accomplice in the event that the person has neglected requirements. For instance, your accomplice might accept you're somewhat far off and may wish that they could invest more energy with you. You really want to know what they need so you can assist with fulfilling their necessities, too.

4. Negotiate with your accomplice: Find shared conviction with your accomplice. This could mean arranging an example of remaining at home occasionally while your accomplice goes out with companions. It could mean welcoming companions over once every month rather than two times per month. Whatever works!

5. Give it an attempt: Implement a thirty-day Challenge. When you think of an understanding, challenge yourself to attempt it for thirty days. Then, see how both of you feel during that period. You may both feel fundamentally more joyful. Then again, a few issues may emerge. In case this occurs, you'll need to make a few changes until you think of a reasonable arrangement that both of you can concur on.

6. Dealing with struggle: Thoughtful people and social butterflies have various methods of taking care of contention. Outgoing people like to face things head-on, and frequently attempt to determine clashes on the spot. Introverts, then again, regularly loathe

contentions. We additionally need time to deal with data prior to responding to questions and settling a contention. To an outgoing individual, it might seem like their withdrawn accomplice is staying away from questions or couldn't care less. As a general rule, the loner just requirements time to think. Additionally, while outgoing people might consider warmed discussions to be important and surprisingly solid, loners might be hesitant to have such discussions since we like "calmer' types of discourse.

Being in a relationship with another introvert

Being involved with an individual thoughtful person may seem like the best circumstance. You ought to have the option to see each other well, and that is significant in any connections. Nonetheless, being with another contemplative person likewise accompanies a few entanglements that you should know of.

- Your mutual desire to avoid conflict may keep one or both of you from bringing up important issues. This, in turn, might make it difficult to move forward in your relationship. You may feel stuck in your comfort zones and unable to take things to the next level.
- You may isolate yourselves from the world. You might get so comfortable spending time alone with your partner that you begin to neglect your social life. We all need to get out and meet other people, no matter how introverted we may be.
- You may rely too heavily on your partner. If you don't have a lot of friends (or you do but don't meet with them often), you may become overly dependent on your partner for your emotional needs.

Raising an extroverted child

For loners, bringing up an outgoing kid can be testing. You might feel overpowered and continually drained. In this segment, I'll offer you some reasonable guidance to assist you with bettering deal with your energy, become a far and away superior parent, and upgrade the nature of your life.

- **Ask your extroverted partner to deal with certain activities:** If your partner is an extrovert, he or she might be able to help you deal with tasks that drain your energy. For example, your partner can deal with most birthday celebrations and talking with other parents. Or they can invest time taking part in outgoing person well disposed exercises with your kid. In the mean time, you're allowed to zero in on errands you can do all alone like cooking or cleaning.
- **Explain to your child that you need your "me" time**: Let your child know that you need some time to recharge your battery. Your child will have to deal with introverts at some point in his or her life, so why not explain what introversion is?
- **Carve out some alone time every day:** Make alone time part of your daily routine.
- **Teach your child to spend time alone:** While introverts enjoy being alone, extroverts crave interaction and may have difficulty being by themselves. You could come up with activities that your child can do alone. Youngster advancement master D. W. Winnicot states that

the capacity to be separated from everyone else "is one of the main indications of development in passionate turn of events." It may be a smart thought to encourage your youngster to invest some energy alone.

- **Reduce your exposure to activities that deplete your energy:** With an extroverted child, it makes sense to reduce any social activities that aren't directly related to your child. Instead of joining group activities, you could choose to have a coffee with a couple of friends, or spend some time alone.
- **Suggest low-key activities you can do with your child**: You could watch a movie or read books together, for instance. I don't recommend you turn your child into a TV addict, but scheduling these types of activities can give you some time to rest.

Avoiding small talk and having deeper conversations

As contemplative people, we pine for significant discussion while keeping away from casual conversation at all costs. For outgoing individuals however, this craving to dive deep so immediately can be viewed as untimely and surprisingly somewhat scary. In this segment, we'll examine how to go further and diminish chatter without terrifying anyone.

1. Be real

Being true from the start is a powerful method for limiting casual banter. If someone says they like something and you don't, then say as much (politely, of course). In case you're worn out, say so. In case you're loathing the party, say as much (pleasantly). By being credible and sharing your musings and feelings, you allow the other individual to do the same.

2. Create hooks by sharing more about yourself

As thoughtful people, we by and large disdain advancing ourselves, yet it's occasionally helpful offer some additional data about yourself. Rather than reacting to, "How are you?" with "I'm fine. I took a stroll in the recreation center close to my home earlier today and the climate was awesome." Or you could say, "I'm extraordinary! I began perusing another book today, and I love it so far."

These little remarks can offer extra ideas to the individual you're addressing. You could even intentionally discard a few subtleties to get the other individual intrigued. In the subsequent model, the other individual may inquire, "What sort of book is it?".

The more you start discussing yourself, the more straightforward it will turn into. You would role be able to play for certain companions or take a stab at adding remarks when you talk with the clerk at the grocery store, for instance.

You can likewise raise a few points you're keen on and attempt to assume responsibility for the discussion immediately. The model with respect to the book you're perusing would be superb assuming you love books and need the discussion to be based on that theme. It will likewise provide you with some try not to try too hardt of what the other individual is keen on. She might cherish writing, science fiction, or books on introspection. Starting there, you can additionally coordinate the discussion. However, though. Ensure it's a two-way discussion and the other individual is keen on the thing you're discussing. Any other way, they'll get bored.

3. Use open-ended questions to deepen the conversation

Asking open-finished inquiries is a powerful method for further developing discussions. The more explicit they are, the better, as they'll give you a brief look into the other individual's reality. Rather than asking what somebody gets a kick out of the chance to do on the ends of the week, for example, ask them what they did this end of the week and what their main thing was. That is the sort of inquiry a companion would ask,
and it can genuinely upgrade the discussion.

Consider asking the accompanying

questions:

- Tell me more about X?
- Are you working on anything exciting these days?
- What was the best part of your weekend?
- What are you looking forward to doing this week?

Obviously, this is only a glimpse of something larger. You can concoct huge loads of other questions!

Asking questions has a subsequent advantage: You don't need to invest as much energy discussing yourself! It will decrease the strain you may feel and make it simpler to support the discussion without becoming anxious.

4. Assume familiarity

When converse with your companions, do you begin the discussion by talking about the climate and asking them how they make ends meet? Obviously not! At the point when you start a discussion with somebody you don't have the foggiest idea, expect commonality and have a go at conversing with that individual as though they were at that point a companion. This implies avoiding standard inquiries with respect to the individual's occupation, old neighborhood, number of kin, etc. As you go further into the discussion, you'll get familiar with the response to those inquiries at any rate. Assuming that you get the ball rolling on a recognizable note, the standard inquiries will be responded to substantially more naturally.

Consider beginning the discussion by asking them how their day was or how they've been doing as of late. You would then be able to begin sharing some data about yourself as we clarified previously. In case the discussion goes no place, you can generally pose less complex inquiries to get things going.

5. Try to learn something

Be interested and enter discussions fully intent on picking up something about the individual you're conversing with. You might even need to move yourself to learn something explicit with regards to them. That will guarantee you're really mindful. It can likewise keep your consideration zeroed in on them rather than yourself.

6. Steer the conversation in the direction of your choice

As contemplative people, we will generally be energetic with regards to specific points. At the point when these subjects are raised, we unexpectedly get invigorated and can't hush up. The good thing is that you don't necessarily have to wait for the topic to be brought up. You can present it yourself and steer the discussion toward the path you'd like it to head in.

You can do this in two distinctive ways:

- **Make a list of your favorite topics:** Then, come up with some stories and questions for each topic. Discussing topics you're passionate about is a great way to see if the other person has similar interests.
- **Come back to something previously said:** You could mention something that they said earlier and ask them to tell you more about it. You could also share your personal experience or opinion on the matter.

An expression of caution:

Don't get carried away. Try not to commandeer the discussion or disregard what the other individual says. If not, they'll get exhausted and quit conversing with you.

Create situations in which small talk is unnecessary

Another method for keeping away from casual conversation is to search out circumstances that don't depend on it. Suppose you choose to join a Meetup bunch encompassing a subject or side interest you're enthusiastic about. Its individuals share a similar enthusiasm or side interest, so casual conversation will turn out to be generally pointless. You can invest your energy discussing your common interests.

Action step

Use the exercise manual (Section III. *Advancing your inner-directedness - 4c. Advancing your relationships)*

- Regarding introversion, what are your biggest struggles in that area? What is one small thing you could do to improve your current situation in that area?

4

LEVERAGING THE GIFT OF INTROVERSION

Introversion accompanies a ton of advantages, none of which ought to be neglected. We want more loners who completely embrace their contemplation and give their gifts to the world. As one of my companions told me, "It's an ideal opportunity to become more friendly, shed the feelings of trepidation, and offer a greater amount of yourself with the world!" That's the message I'd prefer to impart to you. It very well may be the ideal opportunity for you to impart a greater amount of yourself to the world, whatever that means to you.

You weren't conceived a loner to make sure you could profess to be a social butterfly. Would you anticipate that an elephant should climb a tree? You were conceived a self observer, and you're here to utilize every one of your qualities and add to the world however much you can. On the off chance that social butterflies are the yin, thoughtful people are the yang. On the off chance that you invest the vast majority of your energy attempting to act like an outgoing individual, the world will be out of equilibrium for you. Nature and a long period of time of advancement can't be off-base. Assuming loners represent around half of the populace, this is on the grounds that we play a part to play in our society.

Millions of loners before you have utilized their gifts to make the world a superior spot. You can, as well. Presently, how about we turn out a portion of the qualities that are normal in introverts.

Action step

Answer the accompanying inquiry in your exercise manual (Section IV. *Utilizing the endowment of contemplation - 1. Your greatest strength)*

According to you, what is your greatest strength as an introvert?

1. Leveraging your ability to spend time alone

> *I owe everything that I have done to the fact that I am very much at ease being alone.*
>
> — MARILYNNE ROBINSON, NOVELIST AND ESSAYIST.

You might think little of it, however your capacity to be without anyone else is probably your greatest strength. Utilize this time admirably, and you'll accomplish outstanding things in your day to day existence. Your capacity to invest a lot of energy alone doesn't simply permit you to think and concoct good thoughts, it additionally empowers you to get to know yourself on a more profound level. Moreover, your 'alone time' gives freedoms to rehearse your specialty. For outgoing people, investing energy alone doesn't come that easily.

2. Leveraging your propensity for deliberate practice

Practice is the thing that makes champions. It has been shown that specialists invest more energy taking part in what is regularly alluded as intentional practice than a great many people do. For loners, who would prefer to be left alone than work in groups, purposeful practice comes easier.

For example, concentrating on alone utilizing intentional practice has been demonstrated to be the best indicator of expertise for chess players.

Grandmasters, during their initial ten years, go through 5,000 hours concentrating on the game without help from anyone else. This is very nearly multiple times the quantity of hours middle of the road level players spend concentrating on the game. Also, college understudies who study without anyone else will generally learn more than the individuals who work in gatherings. Similar applies to numerous different abilities, sports, and games.

Steve Wozniak, the prime supporter of Apple, credited his introspection for his inventiveness and achievement. He conceded that he couldn't have ever found out such a great amount about PCs assuming he wasn't too withdrawn to even consider going out. He invested a great deal of energy without anyone else finding out with regards to them, not on the grounds that he knew all the science behind conscious practice, but since he was a thoughtful person with a solid enthusiasm. In his journal, he offered the accompanying guidance, "Work alone. You will be best ready to plan progressive items and highlights in case you're chipping away at your own. Not in a board. Not in a group." I think this is valid, particularly for introverts.

What exactly is deliberate practice?

In their book Peak, Secrets from The New Science of Expertise, Anders Ericsson and Robert Pool recommend that purposeful practice:

- Builds skills for which effective training techniques have already been established
- Takes place outside one's comfort zone, requires significant effort, and is generally not enjoyable
- Involves specific, well-defined goals
- Involves taking conscious action and requires a person's full attention
- Involves regular feedback and requires adequate responses to said feedback
- Both creates and relies upon effective mental representation (the patterns we mentioned earlier) and
- Almost always involves working on existing skills or building new ones by focusing specifically on some aspect of those skills that needs to be improved.

It's not difficult to perceive how intentional practice can prompt preferred long haul results over "simply investing the energy." Deliberate practice makes you work both more brilliant and harder by deliberately zeroing in on further developing the abilities you want to come to your goal.

You may be thinking, "In case conscious practice is so extraordinary, for what reason aren't more individuals utilizing it?" There are three primary explanations behind that:

1. Deliberate practice should be founded on existing preparing procedures that are viable. It functions admirably with exercises for which execution can be solidly evaluated, similar to sports, music, or chess. However, it's harder to execute exercises where execution is more hard to survey (like educating or business management).
2. It requires exertion and, let's be honest, the vast majority aren't willing to go through the hassle.
3. Many individuals simply don't be aware of intentional practice and how they can utilize it to work on their skills.

Below are a few instances of what purposeful practice is and is not.

Writing:

<u>Typical practice:</u>

Composing, writing, and seriously composing. In the expressions of Stephen King, "Assuming you need to be an essayist, you should complete two things over all others: read a great deal and compose a ton." But imagine a scenario in which it's more complicated than that?

Deliberate Practice

It appears like Benjamin Franklin felt he expected to accomplish more than peruse and compose a ton. He zeroed in on working on explicit abilities: his composing style, jargon, and feeling of organization.

- Writing style: He made notes on articles from *Spectator*, a high-quality newspaper, which he would use to rewrite the articles a few days later. He would then compare his version to the original and modify it accordingly.
- Vocabulary: He rewrote *Spectator* essays in verse and then in prose so that he could compare his vocabulary to that which the original article used.
- Organization: He wrote summaries of every sentence in a particular article on separate sheets of paper. He would then wait a few weeks prior to moving himself to compose the article aligned correctly contrast his work with the first article.

Doesn't unreasonably seem like fun? Furthermore he did that reliably while holding down an everyday job!

Public speaking

Typical practice:

Practicing a specific discourse over and over until your presentation becomes satisfactory.

Deliberate practice:

Focusing on a particular expertise or part of your discourse that would permit you to work on your general exhibition. These abilities and viewpoints incorporate the following:

- The tone of your voice
- Your rhythm
- The structure of your speech
- Your body language/eye contact
-

- The use of your space
- How you tell stories
- Your vocal projection

As you begin utilizing purposeful practice in your day to day existence, you'll have the option to improve results than the vast majority. Furthermore in spite of the fact that training is best done alone, the advantages of purposeful practice aren't restricted to solo exercises. Public talking, which includes interfacing with a room loaded with individuals, requires a ton of purposeful practice. Nonetheless, you can positively turn into an extraordinary public speaker in the event that you decide to. The equivalent goes for some other abilities you need to create to make the existence you want.

3. Leveraging the time you spend thinking

> *It's not that I'm so smart, it's just that I stay with problems longer.*
>
> — ALBERT EINSTEIN.

As loners, we will more often than not might suspect a great deal. This can be a stunning strength, as believing is the way to critical thinking, and it's been the wellspring of many astounding thoughts and developments. A singular's capacity to remain with a specific subject for an extensive measure of time can yield some magnificent things. All things considered, understand that this strength requires sharpening, any other way it can undoubtedly transform into a weakness.

Sometimes we suspect as much we would even struggle resting. Our capacity to think so strongly can abandon being a gift to a revile assuming we can't handle our musings properly.

While extroverts are often able to take action without thinking excessively, as introverts, we tend to overthink things. If we want to do something, we'll go over it so many times that just *thinking* about what it will involve drains us! *I need to take my car, then I'll have to find a place to park it. The shop will be crowded and I'll get tired. What if they don't have the right size or color. Then, when I'll go home it might be the rush hour etc.* It's almost as draining as actually *doing* what we're *thinking* about. We create all types of scenarios in our minds, which just wastes our precious energy.

Since we exhaust our energy during most friendly associations, this propensity to overthink may be a guard component to secure our energy and try not to take on beyond what we can deal with. That would seem OK. But overdoing it actually *wastes* our energy.

Thinking is one of the most incredible assets we have as people. At the point when we start zeroing in our musings on something critical to us, we begin releasing our loner power.

Since thoughts can be more invigorating for us than whatever else, utilizing our fixation to defeat a specific test can permit us to accomplish incredible results.

Tip: Each time you find yourself overthinking, advise yourself that you can just approach slowly and carefully. At the point when you figure out how to approach slowly and carefully and

quit attempting to anticipate the future, things can turn out to be substantially less overwhelming.

4. Leveraging your ability to stay focused and dig deep

As contemplative people, we for the most part incline toward profundity to expansiveness. We like to dig all the more profoundly into explicit subjects, which can be utilized for our potential benefit. At the point when we observe something we're energetic about, we can get truly energized and extraordinary with regards to it. For example, we might hush up for most of a discussion, possibly to talk constant when a subject of interest comes up. When that occurs, we'll begin talking unquestionably and will be really difficult to quiet down. Does any of this sound natural to you?

Nowadays, many individuals battle to zero in on something particular and on second thought hop starting with one subject then onto the next. Even when they do have a specific goal, they jump from one diet to another, one course to the next, or this book to that book. Then they wonder why they fail to obtain the results they want. This is Shiny Object Syndrome, and it's a significant issue for some individuals. The incredible thing about self preoccupation is that, as I would see it, it makes it more straightforward to stay zeroed in on one objective until it's accomplished. That is on the grounds that self observers are less invigorated by oddity and outer prizes. As Einstein says, "It isn't so much that I'm entirely shrewd, it's simply that I stay with issues longer." The more you train yourself to zero in on one thing you love and go further with it, the more joyful you'll be. This will likewise expand your odds of accomplishing the outcomes you want.

Now that we've covered the absolute most significant qualities that accompany extroversion, it's an ideal opportunity to discuss steadiness. We should get started!

5. Leveraging your writing skills

Many thoughtful people compose better compared to they talk. In that capacity, making a propensity for composing each day can have a major effect in your life. It will assist you with concocting incredible experiences that will help you in numerous spaces of your life.

Keep a journal

Journaling can be useful to anybody, however loners might think that it is particularly useful. Writing every one of your considerations and thoughts down gives two advantages:

1. It permits you to distinguish negative idea examples and restricting beliefs.
2. It helps you in concocting new ideas.

Identify negative thought patterns and limiting beliefs

As contemplative people, we might think excessively. However the key inquiry is what is our take on most? While we have huge number of contemplations consistently, the vast majority of them are similar considerations we had yesterday, last month, or even the year before. Our mind resembles a PC. It runs its own projects and programming dependent on prior convictions. These center convictions are the consequence of rehashed openness to outside upgrade, and they sway our activities on an everyday basis.

As you continue journaling, these center convictions will turn out to be clear. You may continually feel like you're not adequate. Or then again you may understand that specific outside occasions make a specific enthusiastic reaction.

These idea designs are self-maintaining and feed themselves. An outer occasion triggers a center conviction and produces an idea. You consider that idea, which triggers an enthusiastic response. This enthusiastic response thusly supports your idea design.

Model: Someone let you know your discourse might have been something more. You associate this occasion to your center conviction of "I'm not adequate". It produces musings like "I'll never be sufficient" or "I'm moronic". You relate to these musings and trust them, which makes an enthusiastic response. This passionate response could be disgrace, disappointment, or outrage, among other things.

To conquer your prosperity restricting convictions, you should initially distinguish what your writing computer programs is. That is, the thing that your idea designs are, and what triggers them. The more you are familiar yourself, the better you'll have the option to recognize your negative examples and quit engaging pointless considerations. You'll begin considering them to be a messed up record playing a similar tune over and over. You'll become weary of it over the long haul and stop listening.

Each time you experience negative feelings, ask yourself the following:

- What was the trigger? - What made me shift from happiness or neutrality to a negative state of mind?
- What was the exact thought generated by that trigger? - What thought did I identify with?
- How did that make me feel? – Ashamed? Guilty? Frustrated? Angry? Sad? Something else?
- How is it serving me? - Does it serve a purpose? Is it helping me in some way?
- How often have I had similar thoughts in the past? - Is this thought like a broken record? Have you had it thousands of times before? *Use the old entries of your journal and look for similar patterns. What happened in the past?*

After the negative feelings are gone, ask yourself the accompanying three questions:

1. What was the trigger? - What made me shift from a negative perspective to a positive one?
2. What was my manner of thinking? - What thought(s) made that shift?
3. How did this negative influx of feelings serve me? Did I take in something from them, or were they an exercise in futility and energy?

This cycle will assist you with understanding that, more often than not, your negative feelings aren't helping you. That doesn't imply that they fill no need, in any case. Whenever utilized accurately, they can compel you to peer somewhere inside yourself and inspect the center convictions behind these negative feelings. This, obviously, permits you to change your convictions for the better.

Coming up with new ideas

Have you at any point had an extraordinary thought that you ended up neglecting? I have!

Journaling is an incredible method for catching every one of your thoughts in a single spot. It holds you back from failing to remember the creative musings that come your direction. As thoughtful people, we will quite often be imaginative and appreciate pondering different ideas. We feed on thoughts. Thus, the more we catch, the better!

Many of your thoughts will not prompt anything, yet some of the time they can change as long as you can remember. You could think of a thought that transforms into a seven-figure business. You could have a thought for a book that will turn into a blockbuster. Or then again you could have a thought that will totally change the manner in which you see the world.

If you're not journaling yet, why not begin today?

6. Leveraging your interpersonal skills

As a contemplative person, you might be better at talking in little gatherings or having one-on-one discussions. Many contemplative people have great listening abilities that they can use for their potential benefit. Why not use your qualities and focus on circumstances that better suit your character? You'll feel expanded degrees of joy, certainty, and skill, something you can't do on the off chance that you're driving yourself to carry on like an extrovert.

Let's simply say you're searching for a beau or a sweetheart. Certainly, you could go out each end of the week, wear your outgoing individual cap, and pray for divine intervention. But that's likely to leave you tired and frustrated. It presumably will not yield any outcomes, either.

In this situation, why not forget about loud and crowded environments and play the game on your own turf? Wouldn't it be better to be in situations where you can have the kind of conversations you're good at? Putting yourself in favorable situations will give you more opportunities to show your personality.

To this end, you could attempt web based dating. You could likewise go on a twofold date with your companion, or meet individuals in bistros or libraries. You could even join Meetup gatherings to associate with individuals who share your inclinations. You'd be in an ideal situation investing energy with individuals who have comparable interests than waiting around at a party you're not enjoying.

When you spend time with individuals who have comparable interests, it's simpler to start up discussions and casual conversation is superfluous. Actually, I think that it is simpler to interface with individuals when I'm discussing things I love than I do when at a mixed drink party. What about you?

7. Practicing Meditation

Meditation can be especially useful for thoughtful people. In spite of the fact that thoughtful people might appear to be quiet on a superficial level, their internal universes can become tumultuous. Actually, a book can get me so energized I struggle sleeping.

On the other hand, a few of us can suffocate in rushes of negative feelings that require days to get away. I've encountered this myself. I used to scrutinize and even affront myself for not being the individual I needed to be. Reflection permitted me to remove myself from my considerations and quit viewing them so in a serious way. In the midst of stress, reflection has improved my temperament and empowered me to expand my focus.

As such, I ruminate for 25 minutes as a feature of my every day morning ritual*. I urge you to take on a day by day reflection practice, as well. You can begin with just five minutes for every day.

**If you need to make a day by day wake-up routine that upholds your objectives and builds your satisfaction, check out my book* Wake Up Call. *The book will give you a basic, 10-venture strategy you can utilize immediately to make an enduring morning ritual.*

8. Leveraging your ability to persevere

Introverts will quite often remain fixed on an errand longer than outgoing individuals. That is on the grounds that we're less reliant upon outer prizes and moment delight. We needn't bother with that additional surge of dopamine however much social butterflies do. In this manner, we think that it is more straightforward to think long haul and expect potential risks.

Perseverance regularly beats ability. When we can keep up with our degrees of persistence, over the long run, we will actually want to get things done that are a long ways past our minds. Likewise with Einstein, our penchant to "remain longer with issues" can make a major difference.

What if you could leverage your perseverance to achieve your goals and dreams? What if you could use it to create a happier life? This could be done by learning a new skill that allows you to fire your boss and work as a freelancer. And that's just one of the many possibilities!

In this segment, I'll offer a basic strategy to assist you with turning out to be essentially more skilled at persisting and take advantage of your introversion.

Prepare yourself mentally

Many individuals surrender when they understand that things aren't going just as arranged. At the point when they neglect to acquire unmistakable outcomes following a few months, they leap to something different and rehash a similar accomplishing, accomplishing nothing generous. Whatever your objective might be, you'll face many testing circumstances. Truth be told, you're probably going to wind up very nearly stopping many, numerous times.

One of the primary reasons individuals surrender is on the grounds that they start their excursion with unreasonable assumptions. They innocently accept that things will go as arranged, when we as a whole realize that they never do.

To avoid giving up too quickly, it's important to prepare for the worst even before you even start working on your goal. Ask yourself, what's the worst that could happen? What is the worst-case scenario ever? What would you do if you work on your side business for 6 months without making a single sale? What if you can't sell even one copy of that book that took you months or years to write? Considering scenarios like these will serve you well in the coming months. Make sure you visualize the situation and engage your emotions. How would you feel? Could you accept what was happening and keep pushing forward?

Let me give you a new model identified with this book. A brief time prior, the PC I had been utilizing for quite some time smashed and I lost every one of my information. Much more terrible, I hadn't upheld up any of my information (I know, I know…). Therefore, I lost the two new books I was chipping away at alongside numerous different documents identified with my business. The 25,000 words I composed for my self preoccupation book? Gone! Indeed, I needed to modify the book you're perusing right presently without any preparation. What an outright nightmare!

When I envisioned the most dire outcome imaginable, I had imagined losing every one of my books on Amazon and each of the articles on my blog. Anyway improbable, I considered the possibility of Amazon shutting my record for reasons unknown and my site being hacked. The fact wasn't to thought of a reasonable scenario,

however to think of the most noticeably terrible one to set myself up for potential difficulties ahead.

When I lost every one of my information and acknowledged I would need to revamp this book without any preparation, I was unsettled with regards to it. Notwithstanding, I didn't harp on it for quite a long time. I didn't get discouraged and squander a whole week attempting to change the past. I returned to work immediately, on the grounds that I was intellectually ready for it.

Presently, envision what would've occurred assuming I anticipated that things should go flawlessly with practically no difficulties. I would have been crushed, wouldn't I? That is the reason planning for the most noticeably terrible is a savvy thing to do. I hope to experience many difficulties later on that are definitely more testing than this one. All effective individuals have needed to confront significant difficulties, and we will, as well. I recollect Jim Rohn talking about how he lost $250,000 on the grounds that he marked an agreement without understanding it. Essentially he as wellk in his example. I did, too. Now, I try to back up my files!

The subsequent inquiry is, what might make you surrender? When might you say nothing more will be tolerated? By concluding this early, you'll realize that, except if you experience that circumstance, you should continue onward. Furthermore you can generally reevaluate the circumstance. Perhaps, you need to leave your place of employment and search for another that is more loner agreeable. Assuming this is the case, what might make you abandon that objective? Will you surrender following a half year? One year? Two years? After ten prospective employee meetings? Twenty? Thirty?

Stick with one major goal

Having such a large number of objectives is quite possibly the most well-known mistake individuals make when they put out objectives. While having bunches of transient objectives may be alright, it's typically counterproductive with regards to long haul ones. It's far superior to stay with one significant objective and accomplish it than to fiddle with a few major objectives. Doing this forms your self-control muscles and means more prominent outcomes over time.

You might need to utilize this book to work on your connections or update your vocation. Or on the other hand maybe you need to turn out to be better at systems administration and manage parties in a more "benevolent" way. In case you attempt to do everything simultaneously, be that as it may, you'll feel overpowered and neglect to accomplish any of your goals.

You'll improve results by zeroing in on one significant objective during the following, say, thirty days.

Let's say you choose to zero in first on your relationship with your accomplice. When you track down a wonderful equilibrium, you would then be able to continue on the following aspect of your life, like your profession. Please note that this doesn't mean you shouldn't do anything to improve other areas of your life. It simply implies that you should concentrate most of your endeavors towards your one essential goal.

Commit to Your Bullet-Proof Timeframe

The Bullet-Proof Timeframe is an idea that I concocted to assist me with staying patient and adhere to my primary objective. The thought behind it is to provide yourself with a timeframe during which you focus on chipping away at your significant objective. The thought is to make a guarantee to yourself to never surrender before the deadline.

My primary objective is to continue to compose books until I arrive at the cutoff time of my Bullet-Proof Timeframe, which is April eighteenth, 2020 (my 35th birthday celebration). Each time I need to surrender, I advise myself that I have time and I take my concentration back to my objective. I've needed to do this many times.

Below is a passage from my book The One Goal, which sums up the fundamental advantages of executing a Bullet-Proof Timeframe. A Bullet-Proof Timeframe does the following:

- **It forces you to select a goal that matters to you**. Why would you care about some distant deadline two to three years from today if your goal wasn't that important?
- **It reminds you that you have time**. You can step back and look at the bigger picture. As you realize you still have time, persevering becomes less of a challenge.
- **It helps you avoid 'Shiny Object Syndrome'**. You'll stop jumping from one thing to the next if you don't get the results you expected. This is a major trap that derails many people.
- **It gives you the option to give up**. You can give yourself total permission to give up, BUT ONLY once you've reached the deadline. Never before. Here's the mindset you want to adopt: *I can always surrender when I arrive at my cutoff time, so for the time being I will hold tight and keep going.*

I trust that at this point you're persuaded of the advantages of setting a Bullet-Proof Timeframe. It will permit you to turbocharge your determination in every aspect of your life.

Goal-setting crash course for introverts

Let's go over an incredible objective setting strategy. This will help you as you work on updating your life as an introvert.

1. How to set goals

Imagine you could accomplish anything you need and had no impediments at all. What are the objectives that, whenever accomplished, would empower you to be the most joyful self observer conceivable? Record anything that rings a bell without judging it.

2. Select one goal

Select the one objective that, whenever accomplished, would biggestly affect your life. Then, at that point, circle it, since that will be your fundamental goal.

3. Make it SMART

Too regularly, individuals put out objectives that are excessively dubious. With regards to objectives, the more explicit, the better! Along these lines, ensure you utilize the SMART objective strategy, which is clarified below:

SMART stands for:

- **S**pecific: What exactly do you want? What are you trying to achieve?
- **M**easurable: Can you assess the progress towards your goal? How will you know if you've achieved it?
- **A**chievable: Is it achievable? Is the timeframe realistic? Can you put in the effort required despite other responsibilities?
- **R**elevant: Is it in line with your values? Is it exciting to you?
- **T**ime-bound: Do you have a clear deadline for your goal?

4. Break down your goals

If your objective is long haul, separate it into a yearly, month to month, week by week, and surprisingly every day objective. Presently, ask yourself how certain you feel about your capacity to accomplish your objective. On a size of 1 to 10, you need to be at a 7 or 8. Assuming you're underneath this, take a stab at broadening your timetable or making your objective smaller.

5. Implement at least one daily habit to support your goal

Implement one little propensity that moves you towards your objective every day. For example, my objective includes composing books, so I ensure I compose each day regardless. My little objective is to compose somewhere around 500 words each day. That doesn't seem like a lot, yet that is near 200,000 words each year or 1,000,000 words in five years. That is around eight 25,000-word books a year. What's more I for the most part compose in excess of 500 words each day! Your every day propensity will assist you with keeping up with force and support long haul inspiration. Moreover, by keeping each new every day objective little, you'll likewise be less enticed to stall. Make sure to utilize purposeful practice with your day by day habits.

Well, that is the finish of this brief training. If you want to learn more about setting exciting goals, feel free to check my goal-setting book here.

Action step

Take an opportunity to finish the activities in your exercise manual (Section V. *Utilizing the endowment of self preoccupation - sub-areas 2 to 8)*

5

TRANSCENDING YOUR INTROVERSION

> *If you're an introvert, find your flow by using your gifts. You have the power of persistence, the tenacity to solve complex problems, and the clear-sightedness to avoid pitfalls that trip others up. You enjoy relative freedom from the temptations of superficial prizes like money and status. Indeed, your biggest challenge may be to harness your strengths fully. You may be so busy trying to appear like a zestful, reward-sensitive extrovert that you undervalue your own talents, or feel underestimated by those around you. But, when you're focused on a project you care about, you probably find that your energy is boundless.*
>
> — SUSAN CAIN, AUTHOR OF QUIET

You've minimized your qualities for an excessive number of years. You've made a decent attempt to be an outgoing individual you failed to remember who you truly are. Actually you're just about as incredible as any outgoing person. You have qualities most outgoing individuals don't. You can turn into a pioneer and a wellspring of motivation for everybody around you. You don't have to have a go at being the most intense individual in the space to get those things done. Your enthusiasm is your qualities, your thoughts are your weapons, and your tirelessness is a secret jewel standing by to be uncovered. Your composed words have power, and when you talk this is on the grounds that you will say something significant. Over the long run, individuals will figure out how to pay attention to you. Also now and again, unexpectedly, you'll just think of the ideal thing to say.

Obviously, your power will possibly rise to the top when you figure out how to accept your self preoccupation. At the point when you go gaga for quiet. At the point when you quit saying 'sorry' for what your identity is. At the point when you get out of your usual range of familiarity, not really you can attempt to behave like a contemplative person, but since it's what your main goal or your calling expects you to do.

There are numerous fantasies out there That would persuade you to think loners have constraints and can't do what others can. That, notwithstanding, is absolute BS. In case you get tied up with these suppositions, you'll pass up freedoms to uncover your actual potential. Do you know what Nelson Mandela, Mahatma Gandhi, and Mother Theresa shared practically speaking? Indeed, they were incredible pioneers, however there's something different: They were thoughtful people. So how might anybody say thoughtful people can't be pioneers? How might anybody say that we should be fixed? I don't buy both of those assumptions.

During graduate school, I told a cohort of mine that I was keen on instructing. Do you know what she said? "You? You're excessively peaceful. You won't ever talk. How might you Maybe become a mentor?" Taking that idea to is obvious end result, I ought attempt take a stab at nothing since I'm a thoughtful person. Perhaps, I should remain at home and not try to challenge myself. Please accept my apologies, however that is not what's going on with self preoccupation. I don't care for individuals letting me know what I can do and can't do. Do you?

When I ran a study getting some information about their greatest difficulties as self observers, one of the members composed the following:

The most serious issue I see my kindred Introverts encountering is tolerating that they are not odd or faulty on the grounds that they are distinctive in their needs and needs. Likewise, that they can would whatever they like to, regardless of whether it's in the Extrovert world, as long as they make time to really focus on themselves.

He continued:

Despite the reality I've been named an outrageous loner, I had an extremely fruitful vocation in deals which regularly expected addressing enormous gatherings. I cherished my work, I just consistently ensured I put away opportunity to refuel after I must be "on" for a gathering or client.

Did I specify that he was likewise a mentor? Stand by a moment. I figured contemplative people couldn't become mentors. This contemplation thing is certainly more complex

than I used to think!

Finding your passion

It's not difficult to permit yourself to become diverted and wind up consuming your time on earth doing what society anticipates that you should do. My estimate is that you don't need society to tell you to carry on with your life as an outgoing individual, assuming you did, you wouldn't peruse this book, would you?

You likely don't need society to listen for a minute profession you ought to have, all things considered. To flourish as a contemplative person, you should become completely clear on what you need to do. The inquiries beneath will assist you with explaining your enthusiasm. I talked with myself to provide you with an illustration of this exercise.

Who do you begrudge? - This is an incredible inquiry and it ordinarily shows what you are drawn to.

I begrudged self-improvement bloggers like Steve Pavlina and Leo Gura. At some point, as I was watching a video from Leo Gura, everything turned out to be clear. I thought, "This is it." I understood precisely what I needed to do: concentrate on brain science and self-improvement to help other people. That lead me to begin my blog in 2014.

What did you appreciate doing when you were a kid?

When I was a child, maybe seven or eight, I read books the entire day. They were youngsters' books, obviously, yet it was the beginning of my adoration for reading.

What exercises do you chip in for at your present place of employment? What might be said about your past job?

At my first work, I elected to compose month to month articles in Japanese with respect to French culture. I additionally held courses. I discussed the social contrasts among France and Japan in one of these workshops. These two models show both my advantage recorded as a hard copy and my advantage in psychology.

At my past work, I needed to sort out the accepted procedures to support development and the sharing of information. I get it's like how I manage my books: I accumulate information from various sources and put them together.

<u>What subject do you typically get eager to discuss? When was the last time you had an energizing conversation?</u>

I appreciate discussing social contrasts, brain research, and (obviously) self-improvement. The last time I got energized was the point at which I discussed my web-based business with a companion a couple of days ago.

<u>What's your method of adding to the world? - Do you need to motivate? Engage? Teach? Mend? Serve? Make art?</u>

I need to assist individuals with acknowledging what their brains are equipped for accomplishing. I need to give them the apparatuses they need to plan their fantasy life.

<u>According to you, what are your special qualities? - What is it that just you</u> can do?

One of my greatest qualities is my capacity to see the best in others—to see what they could turn into. I regularly have confidence in individuals more than they have faith in themselves. My longing to assist individuals and offer data with them is another strength. At the point when I get amped up for a book or a video, I need to impart it to others. I think that it is disappointing when I can't impart things to other people. I would say my affection for learning is another strength. I love devouring new data and getting a handle on new ideas. Learning is an invigorating, yet endless journey.

What about you? What are you energetic about?

Action step

Use the exercise manual to respond to the inquiries above (Section V. *Rising above your contemplation - 1. Tracking down your enthusiasm)*

Supercharging your passion

The majority of us don't care to be told to behave like outgoing individuals, and we'd love to have the option to accept our contemplation proudly. However, how might it work out in reality to be a contemplative person? We've effectively seen that introspection includes the need to invest energy alone to re-energize our batteries. It includes becoming overwhelmed in noisy conditions with heaps of individuals. It additionally implies attempting to associate with individuals and struggling thinking on the spot.

Yet inner-directedness isn't in this waymething that restricts your potential outcomes and forces imperatives. Indeed, you want time alone to renew your energy, yet beside that, you can would anything you like to do. I don't need you to restrict your potential in light of the presumptions you hold about inner-directedness. If what you're passionate about requires you to do sales, then do it. Loners realize how to tune in and pose the right inquiries, so, in fact, they're regularly extraordinary salesmen. Do you recall what the respondent to my overview said? He composed that he "had an exceptionally effective profession in deals." He's a long way from being the one to focus on. Do you recall Mr. Little? He was an astounding public speaker. You could be, as well, if you so desired.

As self observers, we additionally need to perceive that probably our greatest strength is our capacity to become fixated on something. At the point when we observe something we love and that gives us meaning, we can move heaven and earth. Then again, when we have some work that is unsuitable and disregard the things we love, breaking out of our usual range of familiarity can become impossible.

What about you? Do you consider yourself to be in effect excessively extraordinary? Is it accurate to say that you are fixated on something? I used to accept that I was excessively over the top and I really wanted more adjusts in my life. In all actuality I've been this way for the vast majority of my life. In the first place, it began with books. At the point when I was nearly nothing, I would go through the majority of my days perusing books in my room. Then, I start playing video games. From that point onward, I became fixated on table tennis. In high-school, I would train every day before and after school. Then, there was online gaming. I would in some cases play until 4am during the ends of the week. Obviously, my mom was stressed over me. In school, I became fixated on contemplating. At last, I became fixated on close to home development.

While fixation can be something negative, I've as of late began taking a gander at it from an alternate perspective. I thought, "Imagine a scenario where my fixation is really my greatest strength?" I considered what might occur in the event that I chose to accept it as opposed to quelling it. I considered what might occur assuming I zeroed in completely on something I'm energetic about.

Your own story might be not the same as mine, yet you could possibly identify with it somewhat. The fact of the matter is that your craving to dig further and your need to track down significance in what you do can be an incredibly amazing driver. Truth be told, it could in all likelihood be probably your most noteworthy strength as an introvert.

For these reasons, I think getting away from your usual range of familiarity to make your fantasies a the truth is important for contemplation. It's important for giving your gift to the world. I don't consider it to be attempting to be an outgoing person, however that is only my viewpoint. You don't need to concur with me. In the end, the most important thing is that you live a happy life as an introvert and leave this world with no regrets! I think we can agree on that., can't we?

Once you're grounded in your introspection and zeroed in on your main goal, you can turn into an extraordinary guide to other people. Individuals will begrudge your self-control, concentration, and enthusiasm. Self preoccupation is important for what your identity is, so embrace it. Exemplify it. It's important for what makes 'you,' and nothing on the planet can change that.

Action step

Answer the inquiries in your exercise manual (Section V. *Rising above your self preoccupation. - 2. Supercharging your passion)*

- What skills must you develop to supercharge your passion?

- What things beyond your comfort zone will you need to do to live a meaningful life?

Supercharging your ideas

> *Introverts dislike small talk, but we are fluent in the language of ideas and dreams.*
>
> — MICHAELA CHUNG.

As thoughtful people, we love thoughts. Thoughts are what energize us and make us wake up. Chances are, you have a ton of thoughts you've never imparted to any other individual. You might be perusing one book after another, gathering a tremendous measure of information. Or on the other hand you might invest a great deal of energy thinking and concocting new things.

Writing down bits of knowledge in a diary, or investing time to think all alone are compelling ways of producing more thoughts. Obviously, you may not be enthusiastic about imparting your plans to the world. However, that is important for supercharging our contemplation and sharing our gifts to the world. To this end, I trust it's our obligation to put our thoughts out there. As the late Wayne Dyer said, "Don't bite the dust with the music still in you." If you were to pass on today, what thoughts and tasks would the world pass up in light of the fact that you didn't set out to share them? I would rather not kick the bucket with the music still in me. I need to play my music and perceive what it means for my general surroundings. Don't you?

You can share your thoughts verbally or through composition. It very well may be through workmanship or through your business. Whatever the means might be, impart them as well as could be expected. That is the method for supercharging your contemplation. That is the way you can impart your gifts to the world.

Action step

Answer the inquiries in your exercise manual (Section V. *Rising above your inner-directedness. - 3. Supercharging your ideas)*

- Are you capturing your ideas in an effective way? If not, what could you do to capture them more efficiently?
- Are you sharing your ideas and putting them out there? If not, what could you do to share your thoughts and make a greater commitment to the world?

Understanding introversion is not a label to wear

Once we begin getting inner-directedness, we might feel as we don't have to put forth an attempt any longer. We believe that, since we're withdrawn, we should quit collaborating with individuals, avoid public talking, and remain at home however much as could be expected. These things are not generally evident, however.

Yet it's not difficult to succumb to that and live by our own meaning of inner-directedness. As we referenced before, a significant number of us hold bogus suppositions that don't work well for us. At the point when we mark ourselves as contemplative people, we hazard passing up promising circumstances for development by sticking on to convictions that aren't really true.

I don't accept it's practical to figure we can live as per our vision of introspection constantly. Nor is it to our greatest advantage. Similarly as outgoing people might feel forlorn when they have nobody to go out with, we might end up overpowered at parties we didn't plan, or need, to join in. It would be deluding to say that social butterflies have it simple and carry on with impeccably healthy lifestyles, while thoughtful people are a wreck. We as a whole have our difficulties. Many loners endure forlornness, wishing they could interface with individuals all the more frequently. We as a whole need to manage some degree of discomfort.

I would already be able to hear you shouting, "For what reason are you saying I should carry on like a social butterfly!" Don't stress, that is not what I'm saying. It's dependent upon you whether you need to learn public talking or converse with a many individuals at a party. It doesn't mean you're not a loner, it simply implies you're going past your usual range of familiarity to accomplish something you need. I've tracked down that, when I have a solid feeling of direction, I'm more ready to do things that, as a loner, I regularly wouldn't have any desire to do.

For example, I'm not enthusiastic about sharing data about myself, but rather I do it in my books and recordings. I've likewise been an individual from Toastmasters, a public talking association, for a long time. I found that conveying speeches

and shooting recordings isn't simply terrible. I really began appreciating both, basically on the grounds that I have a greater reason. In case I want to shoot recordings or do workshops to contact more individuals, I'll do precisely that. I actually will not do it constantly. What's more I would be hesitant to do it for a purpose I'm not exactly energetic about.

The last guide I'd like toward commit is that it's not difficult to error bashfulness for self preoccupation, or even dread for inner-directedness. Subsequently, I would urge you to give things a shot and test your own limits. You might wind up appreciating exercises that you could never suspected you'd like.

Action step

Answer the inquiry beneath utilizing your exercise manual (Section V. *Rising above your introspection. - 4. Introspection isn't a mark to wear)*

Could naming yourself as a loner (utilizing your own meaning of contemplation) possibly hurt your development and satisfaction throughout everyday life? Assuming this is the case, how?

Becoming a leader

In a gentle way, you can shake the world.

— MAHATMA GANDHI.

Anyone can be a pioneer. Being a pioneer isn't held for outgoing individuals. In case you affect everyone around you, you're now a pioneer. Assuming that you have command over your own life, you have the stuff to be a pioneer. All things considered, isn't a pioneer somebody who ushers others along a specific way? Furthermore how might you lead individuals on the off chance that they aren't motivated by your activities and the control you have over your life.

Indeed, being a pioneer begins from the inside. Your capacity to control your psyche, body, and demeanor decides your degree of impact. That is not something held for outgoing individuals. Numerous extraordinary pioneers have been self observers. They weren't the most intense in the room, yet their activities talked stronger than their words. To reword Gandhi, they were epitomizing the change they needed to find in the world.

Your capacity to lead individuals and rouse them to change relies upon whether they consider you to be a good example. Can you need to say whether you're a pioneer? Ask yourself, "How have I affected individuals around me?" Have you impacted your accomplice, children, companions, or partners decidedly? Do individuals view at you as a job model?

Introverts can be extraordinary pioneers. We can even outflank social butterflies in specific circumstances. A recent report directed by the Harvard Business Review showed that, when driving outgoing individuals, self observer were more compelling pioneers than social butterflies. The inverse was likewise obvious. Outgoing pioneers outflanked thoughtful ones when it came to driving introverts.

Basically, as a self observer, you can be as skilled a pioneer as any extrovert.

Some successful introverts

Now, we should view some profoundly fruitful contemplative people. You'll see that the absolute best individuals on earth are really thoughtful people. Their self preoccupation might even be one reason they arrived at the apex of success.

Bill Gates - Fiercely un-shy

The organizer of Microsoft can be exceptionally calm, however he turns out to be extremely candid with regards to his energy, which is business. I accept this is valid for some loners. Our enthusiasm can empower us and give us huge power.

Gates said the accompanying in one of his speeches:

> I think introverts can do quite well. If you're clever, you can learn to get the benefits of being an introvert, which might be, say, being willing to go off for a few days and think about a tough problem, read everything you can, push yourself very hard to think out on the edge of that area.

Warren Buffet - Calculated risks

This fruitful financial backer is a contemplative person. His capacity to go ahead with carefully thought out plans of action rather than allowing energy to hold him up is likely essential for his prosperity. While numerous financial backers live close to Wall Street, he resides in a humble house in Omaha, far away from the hype.

Mark Zuckerberg - Depth over breadth

The organizer of Facebook is a loner. He might not have however many associations as outgoing CEOs, yet his capacity to make certifiable associations and convince startup organizers to join his organization is most certainly a strength. As a contemplative person, his longing to focus on profundity over broadness appears to work in his favor.

Fast Company's article "Facebook's Plan to Own Your Phone," had this to say:

> The fact that Zuckerberg can more often than not persuade startup founders to join the company and work with him is a vote for the glass-half-full perspective. 'What I found compelling was Mark's commitment to spending a lot of time with us.'
>
> — BRENDAN IRIBE, OCULUS CEO

Cristina Aguilera - Intensity

You would expect the pop star Christina Aguilera to be an outgoing individual, however she is really a loner. She uncovered to Marie Claire that she had consistently been extreme and thoughtful. She felt like an outcast her entire life.

This demonstrates that nothing keeps thoughtful people from becoming extraordinary performers. Putting on an act or playing a specific person can really be truly pleasant for us. It offers us chances to communicate our thoughts without interference. How cool is that? That is the reason I at times appreciate public talking. I realize individuals need to pay attention to me, and there's a great thing about that.

Emma Watson - The non-party girl

In a world that anticipates that people should act like social butterflies, this entertainer once felt like something wasn't right with her. She would have rather not go out and "have a good time" like her companions. She referenced that finding out with regards to contemplation was a consolation and very empowering.

> " The truth is that I'm genuinely a shy, socially awkward, introverted person," she said. "At a big party, I'm like Bambie in the headlights. It's too much stimulation for me, which is why I end up going to the bathroom! I need time outs! You've seen me at parties … I get anxious. I'm terrible at small talk, and I have a ridiculously short attention span.

Mahatma Gandhi – Thoughtful

Speaking finally was a battle for Gandhi for the duration of his life. Like most self observers, he really wanted chance to set up his talks. He painstakingly picked his words. However that mindfulness saved him numerous problems.

As he said himself:

> " And I can now give myself the certificate that a thoughtless word hardly ever escapes my tongue or pen. I do not recollect ever having had to regret anything in my speech or writing. I have thus been spared many a mishap and waste of time.

Albert Einstein - Staying with problems longer

Einstein, as most contemplative people, did his best reasoning while alone. His capacity to invest energy alone and keep fixed on an issue for a broad timeframe may have added to his revelations. Zeroing in on a particular objective for quite a long time without being diverted has been demonstrated to be a critical component for success.

"It isn't so much that I'm so savvy," he once said. "It's simply that I stay with issues longer."

According to society, you may not wind up as fruitful as individuals I've referenced. However I have almost certainly that you have remarkable space for development. Accepting your introspection rather than considering it to be an impairment will permit you to have an effect in others' lives. The inquiry is, how might you do it? Will it be through your power? Your determination? Your mindfulness? Your fixation on your energy? Your thoughts? That is the thing that you'll need to figure out!

Action step

Answer the inquiries underneath utilizing your exercise manual (Section V. *Rising above your self preoccupation. - 5. Turning into a pioneer)*

- What would you say your biggest strength is? (Thoughtfulness, perseverance, intensity etc.)
- What is one strength, that, if further developed, would make the biggest difference in your life?

Printed in Great Britain
by Amazon

44849819R00047